Alfonso Balmori Martínez

Human ANTENNA

w Atmospheric Changes and Electromagnetic Radiation Affect Us

Anxiety, insomnia, fatigue... It might not be stress. These are invisible forces that disrupt your health —and they're everywhere.

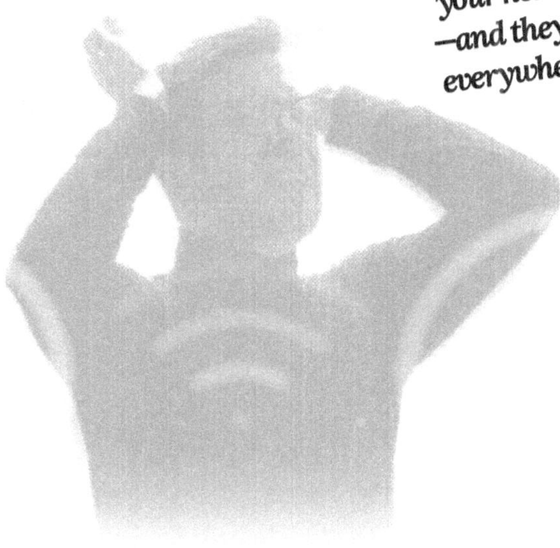

What one generation regards as the pinnacle of knowledge is often deemed absurd by the next, and what is dismissed as superstition in one century may become the foundation of science in the next.

PARACELSO, 1529.

A new scientific truth does not triumph by convincing its opponents and making them see the light, but rather because its opponents eventually die, and a new generation grows up that is familiar with it.

MAX PLANCK, 1947.

www.arcopress.com
@arcopresslibros

www.arcopress.com

Primera edición, mayo 2026

Arcopress • Salud y bienestar
Dirección editorial: Pilar Pimentel

Editorial Almuzara S. L.
Parque Logístico de Córdoba. Ctra. Palma del Río, km 4
C/8, Nave L2, nº 3. 14005 - Córdoba
info@almuzaralibros.com

ISBN: 978-84-10354-79-1
Depósito Legal: CO-777-2026

To my father, who taught me to observe the weather
and has now become part of it.

To my mother, ever cheerful and full of life.

To Mari Paz, Alfonso, José Antonio, and Jaime my steadfast advisers.

To César and Jaime, impervious to discouragement.

In memory of Arthur Firstenberg (1950–2025)
a brave pioneer in the fight against electromagnetic pollution,
with gratitude for his generous mention in The Invisible Rainbow.

INDEX

AUTHOR'S PREFACE

It is striking — and seemingly fortuitous — how similar discomforts can appear simultaneously in different people. How several individuals in the same household may wake up at once with a headache, feel unwell, or find themselves irritable; how, on certain days, schoolchildren seem unusually restless or agitated, while on others an almost absolute calm reigns in the classroom, as if some hidden, mysterious force of nature were at work. These recurring observations raise a legitimate question: can such synchrony truly be due to mere coincidence?

This book seeks to explain how, even in the twenty-first century, we still do not fully understand the extent to which certain little-known elements of nature influence our daily lives — even intruding into our most intimate sensations and emotional states. How the normal circumstances of any person's life are subtly modulated or shaped by unseen forces that may, quite often, affect us in ways more decisive than we imagine.

In this paradoxical era, marked by a widespread sense of superiority over the other species with which we share our journey on planet Earth, we humans might, in some respects, resemble marionettes moved by strange invisible forces that govern our lives far more than we would like to believe.

Human Antennas does not deal with magical or pseudoscientific matters, but rather offers an objective review of what scientific knowledge has so far discovered and demonstrated, in an effort to clarify the foundations of these seemingly inexplicable phenomena. Although some chapters address scientific concepts that may be complex, the aim is for the book to be accessible to a broad readership — to help readers grasp how deeply human beings are embedded within nature itself.

For this reason, the overall tone of the work is informative and approachable. In those chapters that are more technical, or that may evoke a healthy degree of critical skepticism, references to the relevant scientific publications are provided. These are listed alphabetically in the bibliography at the end of the book, allowing interested readers to consult them directly for verification or deeper exploration of the topics discussed.

Throughout several chapters, we also examine the health effects of anthropogenic electromagnetic radiation, as well as the complex relationship between science and economics — a recurring source of tension in environmental disciplines when they collide with powerful human interests. Animals and trees act as essential bioindicators, reflecting the state of the environment we share; their wellbeing or decline reveals the impact of our actions on the balance of the human habitat. For this reason, one chapter is devoted to research conducted on this subject, focusing on species that share our living spaces — such as storks, sparrows, and urban trees.

Biometeorology, the discipline in which much of this book can be situated, builds bridges between fields such as medicine, meteorology, biology, zoology, and physics. We live in a time of great advances across all branches of knowledge — yet they remain highly compartmentalized. Studies that encompass multiple sciences, once characteristic of the great minds of the Renaissance, are now almost impossible to achieve. That is why we increasingly need perspectives that cross the virtual boundaries dividing the sciences (boundaries that, in reality, do not exist in the complex fabric of the world). It is in these “border regions” of knowledge that the seeds — and the future — of major scientific discoveries most likely lie.

1 INTRODUCTION

Spiders appear everywhere, and the flies can't seem to stay still. The neighbor — highly sensitive to changes in the weather — tells us that a migraine kept her awake all night. There's a certain nervous tension in the air. Drivers honk their horns with abandon, and it feels as though words themselves have grown a kind of spiny shell that wounds their recipient without intending to... At last, it seems the rain is beginning. A sense of relief washes over us. The instability has passed, and we feel well again. The spiders retreat to their holes. People open their umbrellas and walk peacefully beneath the rain.

In ancient Greece, during the time of Hippocrates — today regarded as the father of medicine — the influence of certain weather changes or meteorological conditions on specific physiological processes was already recognized. However, it was not until the twentieth century, with the development of physics, physiology, and statistics in particular, that these effects began to be studied in a more methodical and rigorous way. Even today, knowledge remains fragmentary due to the great difficulty involved in such studies, as numerous parameters or variables are at play, and multiple disciplines — traditionally little connected — are involved.

Clinical biometeorology examines the effects of various atmospheric conditions on the human body, whether through biophysical, psychosomatic, or as-yet-unknown mechanisms (Martínez-Carpio, 2003). This author notes that physicians working in emergency services, attending to specific populations — such as the elderly or inmates in correctional facilities — empirically observe that certain types of ailments tend to synchronize at particular times of day, on specific dates, or during certain periods of the year, which, in contexts of limited resources, can overwhelm healthcare services.

Our approach to the problem, based on biology, zoology, meteorology, and our own empirical observations (which we will develop in Chapter 4), aligns fully with the assertions made by Dr. Martínez-Carpio twenty years ago.

The sense of the word *weather* to which we will frequently refer in this book pertains to the state of the atmosphere — that is, to the atmospheric conditions, such as temperature, humidity, pressure, and wind, among others, present at a particular place and time. In contrast, the climate of a region corresponds to the average of these atmospheric conditions recorded over long periods. Weather forecasts deal with the weather, not the climate, and it is precisely these specific atmospheric situations — sometimes referred to as "weather types" — that, as we will explore in detail in the following chapters, exert a significant and still little-understood influence on living beings, particularly on their physiological state and behavior.

In humans, feelings of fatigue or depression alternate with elevated mood and euphoria, as if propelled by some secret, enigmatic force. The ailments and pains of certain chronically ill individuals are intensified by the arrival of cold, rain, or changes in atmospheric pressure. Yet there are individual differences in susceptibility to these factors, particularly to atmospheric electricity.

Biometeorology investigates the changes that occur in living organisms in relation to atmospheric conditions. Weather affects all species, both animal and plant, and of course humans. In rainy years, wild plants reach greater size, and trees tend to grow more, both in girth and height, a pattern recorded in their growth rings that allows us to identify periods most favorable for their development (dendrochronology). Fungi find more favorable conditions for reproduction and dispersal, and certain insects can complete several reproductive cycles (generations) within the same season.

Many animals possess a sensitivity that allows them to detect atmospheric variations signaling impending weather changes. Pressure, temperature, air humidity, wind, and atmospheric electricity, among other factors, influence their behavior. Shepherds know from experience that sheep become restless in response to weather changes, making activities such as shearing or milking more difficult under such circumstances.

When a storm approaches, it is common to observe marked agitation and nervousness in animals such as cats, horses, or flies. In contrast, after the storm passes, a sense of relief and well-being is usually experienced, as the oppressive heat diminishes and the lightning discharges to the Earth release the previously accumulated atmospheric electricity.

Several groups of animals are sensitive to changes in air humidity. Spiders, for example, tend to move more frequently in response to weather changes, possibly due to a hygroscopic effect that causes tension or loosening in their webs as environmental humidity fluctuates. Humidity can also affect the functioning of the wings of certain insects. It is also known that some structures, such as mammal hair, have hygroscopic properties; for this reason, materials like hair, fabrics, or dried intestines have historically been used to predict the weather, since changes in humidity are often accompanied by variations in atmospheric pressure.

When atmospheric humidity rises, especially with the first drops of rain, amphibians leave ponds at dusk to explore areas they avoid under other circumstances, as their skin must remain moist at all times. They wander during the night under these conditions, searching for suitable habitats, and unfortunately, they are often found run over on secondary roads, victims of vehicular traffic. Snails, which may have spent weeks or months secluded in their shells, among grass or under stones enduring the typical summer drought, emerge from their dormancy and glide across surfaces, leaving a mucous trail behind.

Temperature is one of the atmospheric factors that most clearly influences the behavior of living beings: plants, animals, and humans alike. Numerous species seek shelter and undergo winter or summer dormancy, while others are well adapted to the cold through thick layers of fat, hair, or feathers.

The migrations of insects and birds are closely linked to the wind and, consequently, to the spatial distribution of cyclones and anticyclones. Migratory species often take advantage of favorable south winds in spring (for example, when a low-pressure system is located over the nearby Atlantic) to travel to northern breeding regions. In autumn, by contrast, they utilize north winds (for example, when an anticyclone is positioned over the nearby Atlantic) to move south toward wintering areas (figure 1).

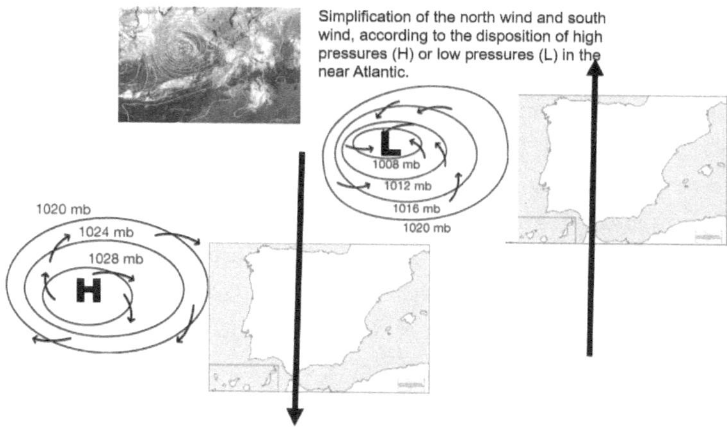

Figure 1: North and south winds, depending on the arrangement of cyclones and anticyclones. An anticyclone is a region of the atmosphere where air pressure is relatively high compared to the surrounding areas. A cyclone is an area of low atmospheric pressure where air tends to rise. In the Northern Hemisphere, winds around anticyclones rotate clockwise, while winds around cyclones rotate counterclockwise (the opposite occurs in the Southern Hemisphere)..

Many species have adapted to prey on migratory birds and insects in the aerial ecosystem, either by capturing birds (such as Eleonora's falcon and the giant noctule) or by taking advantage of migratory moths (such as the European free-tailed bat), whose reproductive cycle shows a bimodal distribution precisely aligned with the spring and autumn migration of these insects (Balmori, 2017).

However, a change in the weather begins to form hundreds of kilometers away from the place where it ultimately manifests. Until recently, it was believed that animals could only anticipate these changes if they were already within the air mass responsible for the phenomenon, and therefore would react only when atmospheric alterations were imminent and locally perceptible. Today, however, we know that electrical discharges generated in cold fronts with associated storms—even hundreds or even thousands of kilometers away—emit electromagnetic impulses that travel at the speed of light and reach great distances. Some people and animals are especially sensitive to these signals, as we will explain in more detail in Chapter 3.

Thanks to this sensitivity, it is not necessary for weather conditions to have already begun changing in a given area to detect the arrival of a distant front, sometimes 24, 48, or more hours in advance, depending on individual sensitivity and other factors that are not yet well understood. For this reason, living beings can anticipate weather changes before they become evident. The hypersensitivity observed in some chronically ill patients—whose symptoms worsen before a weather change—appears to be closely related to the arrival of these invisible electromagnetic impulses. The same applies to certain headaches or migraines, which often precede atmospheric variations.

2
THE INFLUENCE OF WEATHER ON PEOPLE

It is clear that medical science has, to this day, paid little attention to meteoropathies, even though, paradoxically, popular belief—both in everyday conversation and in the doctor's office—may have greatly overstated their importance. It is fascinating to see how some elderly people claim to predict the weather according to how they feel, both physically and emotionally. In telephone consultations with out-of-hospital emergency and urgent care services, peaks in the incidence of certain conditions have been observed—patterns that, so far, very few researchers have shown interest in describing. (MARTÍNEZ-CARPIO, 2003).

Human beings, like all other living species whose life cycles and functions unfold within the Earth's atmosphere, are subject to the influence of weather phenomena. Certain types of weather can bring on ailments, while others provide relief; some cause fatigue or low spirits, whereas others lift the mood or even trigger euphoria.

2.1 Factors to Which These Effects Have Been Attributed

Since the nineteenth century, there have been observations linking certain ailments and diseases to changes in the weather. Yet, despite the time that has passed, a convincing explanation has only recently begun to emerge.

The climatic factors most often considered when exploring or investigating these effects have been the common or easily observable variables—temperature, pressure, humidity, wind, and sunlight. However, to date, although new studies continue to appear confirming some form of relationship, there is still no general consensus regarding which meteorological variable is actually responsible for the symptoms people experience.

We will take a brief look at these more familiar factors, while also introducing some basic concepts necessary for understanding them. These climatic variables undoubtedly produce effects, but they do not anticipate weather changes—that is, they cannot be regarded as their precursors.

2.1.1 Temperature

It is well known that the climate of a given region or country has a notable influence on the temperament and general disposition of its inhabitants. Peoples living in colder areas, where daylight is shorter and less intense, tend to display more melancholic moods, whereas those who live in warmer regions, with longer hours of sunshine, are often described as having a more passionate temperament. Although individuals everywhere may deviate from these broad patterns, certain general tendencies do seem to characterize different populations.

The sensation of cold or heat we experience does not depend solely on the degrees shown by a thermometer at any given moment. Air humidity and wind also play a part, producing very different thermal sensations depending on the circumstances. The feeling of sultriness in humid environments is much greater, just as the perception of cold becomes sharper when accompanied by wind—which strips away the layer of warmth surrounding our bodies—resulting in a thermal sensation or subjective temperature lower than that indicated by the thermometer.

For people, cold and heat limit everyday activities, determine the kind of clothing they wear, and strongly influence the choice of where they live.

2.1.2 Air Masses and Fronts

An air mass is defined as a large body of air—typically more than a thousand kilometres wide and several kilometres deep—that displays almost uniform physical properties, particularly with respect to temperature and humidity. Neighbouring air masses that differ in these characteristics do not usually mix easily; instead, they maintain for some time invisible yet well-defined boundaries. A front, or frontal surface, is precisely the zone of discontinuity that separates two air masses with different temperature and humidity properties. Fronts therefore represent distinct transitions in the characteristics of the air.

Although several types of fronts exist, we will focus here on the two simplest ones: warm fronts and cold fronts.

A warm front separates two air masses—one warm and one cold. The warmer air glides over the colder air mass and, as it rises, gives rise to stratiform clouds (see Figure 2). In contrast, in a cold front, the colder air mass pushes the warmer one upwards rapidly, generating vertically developed clouds such as cumulus formations.

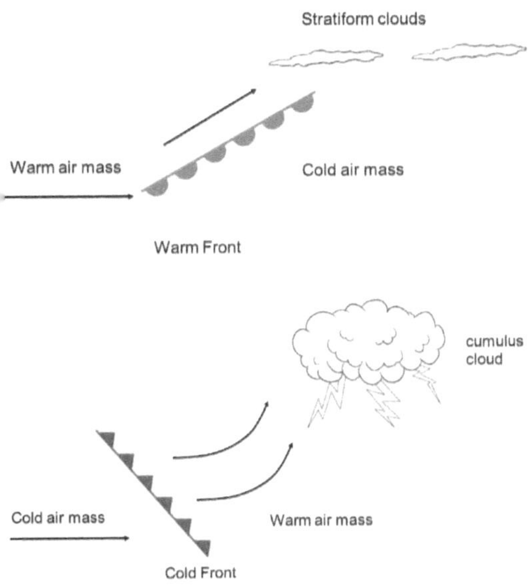

Figure 2. Formation of a warm front and a cold front. Warm fronts are usually represented on weather maps with semispheres and cold fronts with a line of triangles

Later on (in Chapter 3), we will examine in detail the importance of these cold fronts in explaining the ability of living beings to perceive and anticipate weather changes over great distances — often long before these changes reach the place where the animals are located.

Likewise, in the following chapters we will explore the fundamental role of fronts and atmospheric instability in the development of certain ailments or mood states, which often subside after the front has passed, generally leaving behind a sense of well-being. More sensitive individuals, who suffer from what is known as meteoropathy, may experience anxiety or nervousness without any apparent cause. Headaches, rheumatic pain, discomfort in scars and old fractures, as well as epileptic episodes and even heart attacks, may all become more frequent or intense. Moreover, peaks have been observed in both birth and death rates, influenced not only by atmospheric conditions but also by extraplanetary factors—such as solar eruptions and cosmic radiation—which trigger associated geomagnetic disturbances (as will be discussed in Chapters 8 and 9).

These effects are also reflected in people's emotional state, generating feelings of euphoria, depression, or irritability, which in turn affect their efficiency and work performance. For this reason, weather conditions and the various states of the atmosphere acquire considerable significance in business productivity and, consequently, in the economy of nations (Mackensen *et al.*, 2005).

2.1.3 Wind

Wind is usually associated with situations of atmospheric instability and, depending on its direction and speed—as well as the temperature and humidity of the air—it can influence both mental state and physical health.

In each region, inhabitants give specific names to the types of wind that display distinctive characteristics. Some examples include the cierzo in the Ebro Valley, the levante in Cádiz, the tramontana in Ampurdán, the *sharaw* in Israel, the *chinook* in Canada, the *harmattan* in the sub-Saharan region, the *foehn* in Switzerland and Austria, and the mistral in the French Provence.

In northern Spain and southern France, southerly winds are said to cause restlessness and headaches. The *sirocco* of North Africa and the southern Canary Islands is a dry, hot wind that produces fatigue, discomfort, and distress.

The *foehn* wind, characteristic of the northern Alps, is associated with changes in atmospheric electricity and is believed to bring about certain alterations in human behaviour—such as irritability, lack of concentration, headaches, traffic accidents, street fights, and workplace or family disputes (Martínez-Carpio, 2003).

The well-known «foehn effect» owes its name to a particular type of wind that forms when an air mass encounters a mountain barrier—such as a range or a ridge—and is forced to rise. As it ascends, the air cools and the water vapour it contains condenses, giving rise to precipitation. Upon crossing the summit and descending the leeward slope, the air has already lost much of its moisture and becomes a warm, dry mass. Consequently, the windward side, where rainfall occurs, tends to have a humid environment and abundant vegetation, whereas the leeward slope is drier, with generally clear and warm weather.

This contrast between slopes with opposite humidity conditions is common in many mountainous regions and is further accentuated by geographical orientation: in the Northern Hemisphere, north-facing slopes are typically more humid and receive less sunlight than south-facing ones, while in the Southern Hemisphere the opposite occurs.

2.1.4 Storms and Rain

Storms can cause distress in individuals who have had negative experiences in the past, particularly during childhood. They often occur following episodes of sultriness and, once they pass, produce a kind of physical and emotional release. In later chapters, we will examine the significance of storms—especially those associated with cold fronts—in generating electromagnetic radiation in the atmosphere and, consequently, in the ability of sensitive humans and animals to anticipate weather changes.

Rain, on the other hand, tends to foster low spirits and evokes feelings of nostalgia in many people by triggering memories of the past. Among its more tangible effects are an increase in traffic accidents in cities and on roads, as well as various inconveniences caused by the disruption it can bring.

2.1.5 Fog

Like rain, fog is generally associated with low mood in individuals prone to melancholy, as well as with various rheumatic ailments, possibly linked to the high ambient humidity. It also creates conditions of reduced visibility, which can pose risks, particularly for road traffic. In foggy conditions, birds are also at greater risk of colliding with man-made structures such as wind turbines, power lines, and telecommunications antennas.

2.2 Biometeorology: A Bridging Discipline

In 1997, Peter Höppe, a researcher at the University of Munich, published a review in the scientific journal *International Journal of Biometeorology* on the past, present, and future of human biometeorology (Höppe, 1997). This discipline, considered a branch of science closely linked to meteorology and environmental medicine, studies the influence of the atmospheric environment on human beings. It is a fascinating field due to its interdisciplinary nature, although it is also complex and, at times, frustrating because of its inherent difficulties.

Biometeorology developed particularly in Germany, where researchers described how specific atmospheric conditions can trigger distinct patterns of symptoms, known as meteoropathies or hypersensitivity to weather conditions. Closely related to ecology, this discipline analyses the effects of the physical environment—particularly the natural atmosphere (temperature, humidity, barometric pressure, wind speed, air ionisation, sunshine, etc.)—on living organisms (Da Luigi *et al.*, 2013).

Various studies in this field have identified correlations between certain weather conditions and the onset or exacerbation of symptoms and diseases under specific meteorological circumstances.

2.3 Meteoropathy: A Strange Ailment of Unknown Aetiology, Yet All Too Common in the Population

In 2010, W. J. Becker, a researcher from the Department of Neurology at Calgary Hospital (Canada), published an editorial in the scientific journal *Cephalalgia* with a highly evocative title: "Weather and Migraines: Can So Many Patients Be Wrong?" (Becker, 2010).

The term meteoropathy refers to any psycho-organic disorder associated with meteorological phenomena (Martínez-Carpio, 2003). It designates a group of conditions or pathologies that are triggered, activated, or worsened under specific weather conditions.

Evidence is steadily accumulating regarding the interaction between periodic variations in meteorological factors and biological systems. An epidemiological survey-based study on the prevalence of meteoropathic symptoms revealed that in Germany, 54% of the population consider themselves in some way sensitive to weather conditions, while in Canada the figure rises to 61% (Mackensen *et al.*, 2005).

Meteoropathy encompasses a set of symptoms and pathological reactions that manifest in response to gradual or sudden changes in the weather conditions of a particular region (Da Luigi *et al.*, 2013). In general terms, a stable atmosphere dominated by an anticyclone is considered less likely to provoke meteoropathic reactions, in contrast with an unstable atmosphere, especially when abrupt variations in meteorological parameters occur.

In continental Europe, after a spell of fair weather, when a disturbance approaches from the Atlantic (around 24–48 hours before a depression arrives), various effects on the human body can be observed (see Chapter 4). Particularly sensitive individuals may display a collection of symptoms forming the so-called meteoropathic syndrome, especially when several atmospheric factors change simultaneously (Da Luigi *et al.*, 2013).

The most common meteoropathic symptoms include mood alterations, weakness, hypertension, headaches, rheumatic pain, cardiovascular disease, arthritis, hyperthyroidism, stress, anxiety, irritability, neurological disturbances, migraines, epileptic seizures, exacerbation of asthma, and fluctuations in blood glucose levels, among others. These symptoms generally last one or two days, coinciding with the local weather change, only to recur when another shift in conditions takes place. When weather changes occur in succession, a gradual process of adaptation seems to develop, leading to a reduction or disappearance of symptoms.

To this day, most meteoropathic problems or symptoms are attributed to the best-known and most easily measurable atmospheric variables — pressure, wind, temperature, light intensity and duration, humidity, and a higher concentration of positive ions in the atmosphere. However, there is another causal factor, almost unknown yet extremely important, which will be discussed in detail in the next chapter.

For many years it has also been recognised that atmospheric situations and weather changes exert an impact on mood and behaviour that overlaps with the effects of daily life events (problems or joys, successes or failures). Thus, our behaviour is, at least in part, also a result of the physical characteristics of our environment, which stimulate or modulate our organism. Evidence indicates an alternating activation pattern of the sympathetic and parasympathetic nervous systems corresponding to changing weather conditions, which in turn brings about secondary behavioural changes (Persinger, 1980).

Meteoropathic symptoms, which tend to intensify as weather changes approach, are usually more evident and persistent in individuals suffering from anxiety, depression, or neurological disorders. Nowadays, this psychological instability is further aggravated by an increase in negative factors in daily life, such as stress, difficulties in entering the labour market, intense competition, and atmospheric pollution (Da Luigi *et al.*, 2013). Specific questionnaires are currently available to validate the presence of meteoropathy in individuals (Mazza *et al.*, 2012).

Interestingly, the symptoms described in people suffering from meteoropathy closely resemble those observed in patients with electrohypersensitivity (EHS) — a coincidence that is undoubtedly not accidental, as will be discussed in greater detail in Chapter 5.

Although meteorosensitive individuals have always existed, meteoropathy has become increasingly common in recent times, probably caused or exacerbated by modern lifestyles. Middle-aged people (and particularly women) appear to be at higher risk of becoming meteoropaths. Spending too much time indoors or in climate-controlled environments reduces our ability to cope with weather changes and atmospheric conditions in general. Physically active people who spend several hours a day outdoors rarely even notice weather changes. Older adults, however — especially those who remain indoors — feel and suffer every shift in the weather, whether gradual or abrupt.

Several types of meteoropathy have been identified, and their frequency appears to be increasing, particularly in countries where consumer and welfare societies predominate. This phenomenon has been linked to a progressive decline in the body's resilience and immune response (Balsamo *et al.*, 1992). A growing number of people experience the effects of weather changes, which has generated increasing interest in the study and understanding of meteoropathy.

In addition to the involvement of hormonal systems and neurotransmitters, clinical observations suggest that environmental stimuli — especially physical variables — may play a significant role in the complex pathogenic mechanisms underlying psychiatric disorders (Da Luigi *et al.*, 2013).

Martínez-Carpio (2003) argues that the influence of meteorological factors on brain neurotransmitters plays a crucial role in the aetiopathogenesis of many meteoropathies. Likewise, in the field of psychology, various epidemiological studies have demonstrated that, depending on the degree of an individual's meteorosensitivity, mood, pain perception, psychiatric decompensation, suicide attempts, and certain criminal behaviours may all be associated with meteorological variables, which modulate their thresholds of expression to a greater or lesser extent.

Climatic patterns result from a complex interaction among multiple meteorological variables, making their analysis difficult. So far, conventional statistical methods have not proved sufficiently effective in studying these relationships. However, a few years ago, a team of researchers in Taiwan separately analysed the temporal relationship between the onset of headaches and various variables — such as atmospheric pressure, humidity, temperature, and wind speed — under different weather conditions, using a novel statistical approach (Yang *et al.*, 2011). Their results revealed that the approach of cold fronts showed the most significant correlation with the symptoms recorded — a relevant finding that supports the hypothesis to be developed in the next chapter.

3

INVISIBLE MESSENGERS: THE *SFERICS*

In this chapter, we will delve deeper into the specific origin of the symptoms that precede weather changes, as well as into the formulation of plausible mechanisms that may provide a scientific explanation for these phenomena.

Living organisms are continuously exposed to the influence of natural electromagnetic radiation, which spans a wide range of frequencies and amplitudes. It has now been established that, under certain atmospheric conditions (or "weather types"), extremely short yet far-reaching electromagnetic impulses are generated from atmospheric electrical discharges (commonly known as lightning) during thunderstorms. These electromagnetic radiation impulses produced by lightning are referred to as *atmospherics*, VLF-*atmospherics*, or VLF-*sferics*. In what follows, we shall use the shorter and internationally accepted term *sferics*. These *sferics* can be detected and recorded using specialised receiver equipment.

Sferics originate from the enormous voltage differences produced by the exchange of electrical charges between clouds; between clouds and atmospheric particles; or between clouds and the Earth's or sea's surface. When this potential difference reaches sufficiently high levels and, simultaneously, atmospheric conductivity increases—particularly during storms—conditions become favourable for the generation of electrical discharges. These discharges, known as lightning, act as a mechanism of neutralisation, suddenly transferring electrical charge and generating highly intense currents.

The electromagnetic waves generated by lightning (*sferics*) are reflected both by the lower ionosphere and by the Earth's surface, propagating through the atmosphere. This propagation occurs within the space between the Earth and the ionosphere, which acts as a natural waveguide for electromagnetic radiation—a kind of "highway" that facilitates its transmission—, as will be explained in greater detail in Chapter 4.

From a meteorological perspective, variations in the reception of electromagnetic waves generated by atmospheric discharges—detected using appropriate receivers, such as antennas—can serve as early predictors of forthcoming weather changes in a given region. This is particularly valuable when other conventional indicators, such as variations in temperature, atmospheric pressure, or humidity, have not yet become apparent. This predictive capacity arises from the fact that weather fronts move at speeds of tens of kilometres per hour, whereas the *sferics* associated with them travel at the speed of light, enabling these electromagnetic impulses to reach the affected area well in advance.

These electromagnetic radiations affect both the inanimate environment and living organisms. Consequently, in addition to serving as indicators of thunderstorm activity, the electromagnetic impulses generated by lightning can also be perceived by animals, including humans. It is thought that such impulses may act as triggers for changes in somatic and emotional wellbeing—a phenomenon known as "weather sensitivity" or "meteoropathy" (Schienle *et al.*, 2006; Da Luigi *et al.*, 2013).

3.1 Pioneer Authors

The German researchers Hans Baumer and Walter Sönning, two leading specialists in this field, published in 2002 a book that reviews the scientific knowledge accumulated in a discipline developed throughout the twentieth century—primarily in Germany—dedicated specifically to naturally generated atmospheric *sferics*, their effects on living organisms, and their usefulness as meteorological predictors (Baumer & Sönning, 2002). The authors concisely summarise the results of their research carried out between 1978 and 1996, documented in more than fifty specialised scientific publications, and discuss extensively the implications of low-frequency pulses and their biological impact.

They also draw attention to the pressing need for interdisciplinary work involving researchers specialised in neurology, brain physiology, biochemistry, molecular biology, and biophysics—an approach they regard as essential for studying in depth the influence of meteorological factors on biological systems.

Although the evidence for the physiological and organic effects of *sferics* on living beings was steadily confirmed throughout their investigations, it has not yet been recognised or accepted by what they call the "official doctrine". According to the authors themselves, this is due to a kind of scientific inertia and to the habitual tendency to focus research on conventional meteorological parameters—better known, more accessible, and more easily measurable—as already mentioned earlier. In this respect, Baumer and Sönning argue that the biotropic or bioactive factor—whose existence has long been sought in the relationship between living organisms and the atmospheric environment—is not to be found among any of the traditional atmospheric variables, but rather in the *sferics*, that is, in the natural electromagnetic impulses generated within the atmosphere (see Figure 3).

As we shall see in greater detail later on, *sferics* contain sufficient informational content to activate the action potentials of the nervous system, altering membrane permeability and thereby influencing the influx or efflux of specific ions across cell membranes.

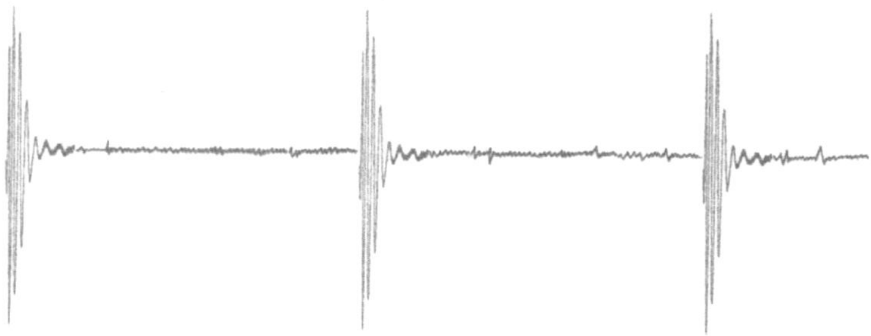

Figure 3. Representation of the typical sferic waveform showing the low-frequency pulses.

The German researchers also explain that *sferics* may exert opposite or antagonistic effects on living organisms, depending on their frequency—particularly within the 10 kHz and 28 kHz range. This variability could account for the abundance of documented examples in the scientific literature describing contradictory effects of low-frequency electromagnetic pulses on living organisms, as observed in laboratory experiments (Brezowsky, 1965; Persinger, 1974).

3.2 The Significance of Sferics

Weather changes begin to take shape hundreds of kilometres away from any given location and, in general, only become clearly apparent in local atmospheric conditions shortly before they occur. These changes first affect the upper layers of the atmosphere. However, between 48 and 72 hours prior to the arrival of a weather front, certain invisible electromagnetic signals —known as *sferics*— can already be detected, heralding its approach. These signals arrive earlier because they travel at the speed of light, which makes it possible to use them as early indicators for weather prediction.

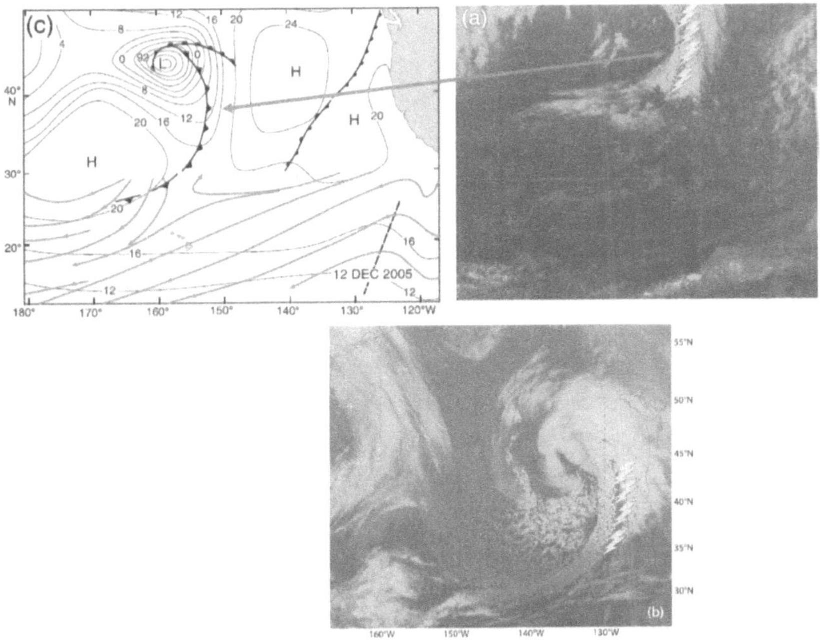

Figure 4. Association of low-pressure systems and cold fronts with increased thunderstorm and lightning activity. Images taken and adapted from Pessi and Businger (2009), with the authors' explicit permission.

The approach of weather fronts—and in particular cold fronts, which are associated with the highest concentration of storms—is accompanied by what could be described as a veritable invasion of *sferics* in the atmosphere, as though heralding the arrival of an invisible battalion.

In the regions where cold and warm fronts originate, turbulent air currents with both horizontal and vertical components are generated thermodynamically. Most lightning activity is associated with thunderstorms, and specifically with convection along cold fronts (see Figure 4). It is here, essentially, that the impulses of natural electromagnetic radiation in the atmosphere (*sferics*) are produced. Frontal systems and moving air masses transmit these signals within the approximate range of 1 kHz to 100 kHz (VLF: very low frequency), which are pulsed (in bursts, see Figure 3) within the ELF range (extremely low frequency), at an average frequency of about 7.5 Hz. Consequently, the thunderstorms associated with these fronts generate *sferics* that travel at the speed of light. These natural electromagnetic pulses can easily be heard on radio receivers as sudden bursts of interference, since their frequencies overlap to some extent with those of man-made radio waves.

The natural ELF signals of the atmosphere originate from the electromagnetic energy released by the thousands of thunderstorms—and the associated lightning strikes—constantly occurring across the planet. This energy is channelled around the Earth and propagates within the space between the Earth's surface and the ionosphere (see Chapter 4), in much the same way as man-made radio waves. The result of this continuous electromagnetic "background noise", generated by the rapid propagation of oscillations induced by thousands of lightning discharges, is a global resonance known as the Schumann resonance, named after the researcher who discovered it. Its fundamental frequency is 7.8 Hz, with harmonics at 14.1, 20.3, 26.4, and 32.5 Hz. All living organisms on Earth are adapted to these frequencies, which gives them great biological significance, as will be discussed later (Chapter 5).

Given that *sferics* propagate from a meteorological front at the speed of light and can travel hundreds or even thousands of kilometres, these signals function as a recognisable meteorological code for animals equipped with the appropriate reception systems. In this way, they can anticipate approaching weather changes, thanks to the volume of electrical impulses detected long before conventional meteorological parameters begin to vary. Various forms of life—such as insects, amphibians, and birds—react to these electromagnetic impulses generated by atmospheric activity. By receiving and interpreting the frequency of these "weather codes", which act as genuine warning signals of meteorological change or approaching storms, they can take shelter or fly away in time to avoid them—an efficient biological strategy (Warnke, 2007).

The particular sensitivity of bees to weather changes is well known and is thought to be based mainly on electromagnetic information.

Mammals and humans are also sensitive to weather changes, owing to our capacity to perceive these electromagnetic impulses (*sferics*) either unconsciously or inadvertently.

The link between weather changes and rheumatic pain is the most commonly reported, given the widespread recognition of such cases in society. Many people suffering from rheumatic pain are able to predict atmospheric changes when their pain intensifies. Moreover, frontal weather systems influence emotional state: as a front approaches, many individuals report feeling disturbed, restless, or irritable. Despite the methodological challenges inherent to questionnaire-based statistical and epidemiological studies, the patients' perception of approaching weather changes remains a difficult fact to dispute (Becker, 2011).

Numerous researchers have examined the association between atmospheric radiation and various health disorders, including certain types of headache, joint pain, epileptic seizures, depressive states, and even more severe phenomena such as increases in suicide rates. Many patients experience crises of varying intensity as meteorological fronts approach, suggesting a particular sensitivity of the organism to changes in the atmospheric electromagnetic environment.

Pain associated with amputated limbs and brain injuries has also been linked to the presence of *sferics*, both in laboratory studies and in field observations. The pioneering work of the German researcher Reinhold Reiter includes references to the aggravation of various pathologies—such as bronchial asthma, circulatory and cardiac disorders, insomnia, headaches, glaucoma, biliary and urinary colic, myocardial infarction, and cerebrovascular accidents—correlated with *sferic* activity (Reiter, 1960). Reiter maintained that *sferics* are good indicators of meteorological change and tropospheric instability (the troposphere being the lowest layer of the Earth's atmosphere, in contact with the planet's surface, roughly 10 kilometres thick, where all meteorological processes occur). In one of his studies, Reiter recorded the frequency of headaches in 120 patients over a 200-day period and found a significant correlation between pain intensity and the number of electromagnetic impulses present in the atmosphere. He also observed a statistically relevant relationship between very low frequency (ELF) electromagnetic wave activity and the average reaction times of exposed individuals (cited in Warnke, 2007).

The approach of a cold front, accompanied by high atmospheric instability, causes a considerable increase in epileptic seizures (Baumer & Sönning, 2002). Patients suffering from pain in scars often perceive the approach of such fronts recurrently. Embolisms, strokes, and myocardial infarctions also occur more frequently with the arrival of weather fronts (Kveton, 1991).

A positive correlation has been documented between *sferic* activity—both in terms of the number of pulses per minute and the intensity of the recorded impulses—and the occurrence of sleep disturbances, errors in tasks requiring concentration, and alterations in the alpha and beta wave rhythms of the electroencephalogram (EEG). These effects can be observed even at great distances—up to thousands of kilometres—from the regions where thunderstorms originate. It is estimated that between 30% and 78% of people who suffer from headaches are sensitive to atmospheric changes, and more specifically to the intensity and frequency of lightning discharges detected per minute. This relationship shows a statistically significant connection (Walach *et al.*, 2001).

In a survey-based study, 54% of Germans and 61% of Canadians reported that their health was affected by weather conditions (von Mackensen *et al.*, 2005). The most frequent symptoms among the German population were headache/migraine (61%), apathy (47%), sleep disorders (46%), fatigue (42%), joint pain (40%), irritability (31%), depression (27%), dizziness (26%), concentration problems (26%), and pain in scars (23%) (von Mackensen *et al.*, 2005).

Sferic activity has been found to correlate significantly with the occurrence of migraines, with 59% of women reporting headaches prior to a change in the weather (Vaitl *et al.*, 2001). This correlation between migraine-type headaches and lightning has been confirmed more recently (Martin *et al.*, 2013).

Furthermore, it has been shown that electromagnetic pulses generated artificially in the laboratory, when exhibiting characteristics similar to atmospheric discharges (*sferics*), affect the human electroencephalogram (EEG), particularly in the alpha (8–13 Hz) and beta (13–30 Hz) frequency bands. Individuals with greater meteoropathic sensitivity and more intense and prolonged pain displayed sustained EEG changes and described the artificial exposure as more exhausting and emotionally distressing (Schienle *et al.*, 2001).

In addition, electromagnetic oscillations generated by charge exchanges in frontal regions of the atmosphere (*sferics*) produce a marked increase in platelet adhesion. It has been observed that individuals with mental instability are more vulnerable to these changes in platelet adhesiveness than those with greater emotional stability. In a controlled laboratory study, platelet adhesion was measured using a sferic simulator. The results showed a highly significant increase ($p < 0.0005$) in platelet adhesiveness when a carrier frequency of 10 kHz with a pulse repetition frequency of 10 Hz (equivalent to 10 pulses per second, within the biologically active "window") was applied. In contrast, platelet adhesiveness decreased when the pulse repetition frequency was 2.5 Hz or 20 Hz (Jacobi *et al.*, 1977).

3.3 Mode of Action of Sferics on Living Cells

So far, we have seen that the electrical discharges occurring during thunderstorms generate electromagnetic impulses known as *sferics*, which can be inadvertently detected by humans and animals at considerable distances from cold fronts, manifesting through various symptoms. However, until quite recently, no biophysical mechanism had been identified to explain how these *sferics* exert their biological effects

In 2017, the Greek researcher Dimitris Panagopoulos and the author of this book published a paper in the scientific journal *Science of the Total Environment*, in which we proposed, for the first time, a plausible explanation for the biophysical mechanisms underlying the capacity of living organisms—and humans in particular—to detect atmospheric discharges (*sferics*) (Panagopoulos and Balmori, 2017).

As is known, *sferics* are partially polarised electromagnetic pulses with an oscillating carrier signal in the very low frequency (VLF) band, and a pulse repetition rate in the extremely low frequency (ELF) band. Their ELF intensity can reach approximately 0.5 V/m at a distance of around 1,000 km from the lightning strike. Most cation channels (Ca^{2+}, K^+, Na^+, etc.) present in the membranes of all animal cells open and close depending on changes in the potential difference between the interior and exterior of the cell and are therefore electrosensitive (Alberts *et al.*, 1994).

According to the biophysical mechanism proposed for the action of oscillating electric fields on cells (Panagopoulos *et al.*, 2000), polarised ELF electromagnetic fields, even of intensities as low as 0.1–1 mV/m, can disrupt the electrochemical balance and function of any living cell by irregularly activating the electrosensitive ion channels in the cell membranes, thereby triggering a range of symptoms and health problems (Panagopoulos *et al.*, 2025). (For a more detailed explanation, see also Section 8.2.)

The heightened sensitivity of living organisms to low-frequency pulsed electromagnetic fields (ELF) can be explained by the physics and biology of voltage-gated cation channels in cell membranes. These waves have a greater capacity to irregularly close such channels, thereby disturbing the electrochemical equilibrium both at the cellular level and within the organism as a whole.

Sferics travel long distances at the speed of light with only slight attenuation, especially within the low-frequency (ELF) band. Could it therefore be possible that partially polarised *sferics* might be detected by living organisms thousands of kilometres away from a thunderstorm? The answer appears to be an unequivocal yes (Panagopoulos and Balmori, 2017).

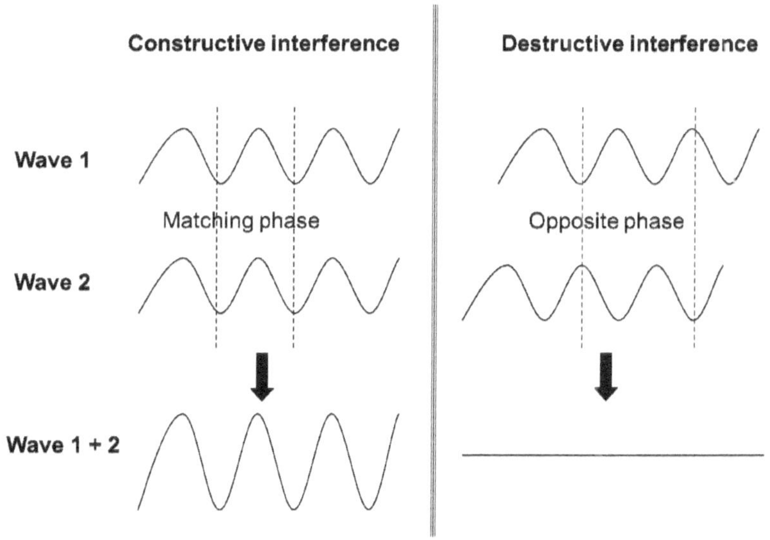

Figure 5. Illustration of constructive and destructive interference, depending respectively on whether the phases of two waves coincide or oppose each other.

On the other hand, simultaneous atmospheric discharges with similar characteristics can create transient constructive phenomena (interferences or couplings), and at such points, living organisms may be momentarily exposed to higher field intensities than those produced by single discharges (Figure 5).

Previously, Panagopoulos, Johansson, and Carlo (2015) published an article in the prestigious journal *Scientific Reports*, in which they explained that polarisation is the key difference between man-made (polarised) electromagnetic fields and natural ones (which are generally unpolarised). This property (Figure 6) is what accounts for the biological activity of so-called "technological" radiation (see Chapter 5). However, although *sferics* are natural atmospheric discharges, they consist of partially polarised electromagnetic pulses of sufficient intensity to produce biological effects, mainly within the ELF band (Panagopoulos and Balmori, 2017). Indeed, they may even generate the same health effects in humans as anthropogenic electromagnetic pulses (see Chapter 5).

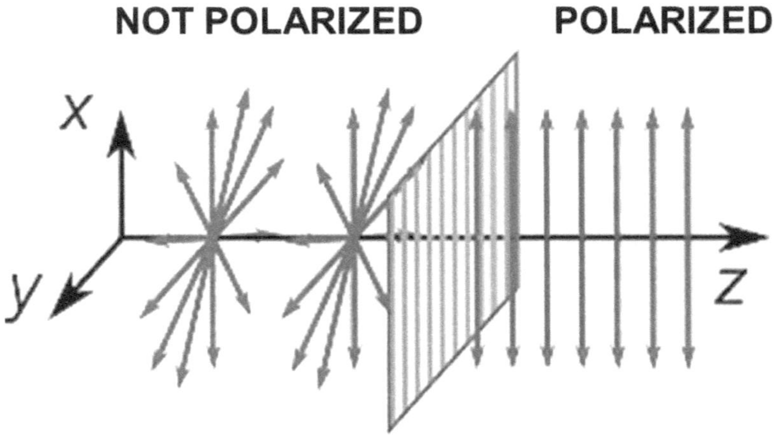

Figure 6. Polarised waves: as the wave passes through the polariser, it changes from vibrating in all spatial directions to vibrating in a single direction.

If the hypothesis we are proposing is correct, meteoropathy (sensitivity to weather changes) and EHS (electrohypersensitivity) would represent two sides of the same phenomenon. The former (meteoropathy) would have its origin in natural electromagnetic radiation, whereas the latter (electrohypersensitivity) would stem from artificial, technological or anthropogenic radiation. In this way, the problem becomes convergent: people with EHS would also be sensitive to natural *sferics*, while those with meteoropathy would likewise be sensitive to technological electromagnetic fields. And this is precisely what is increasingly being observed in the everyday reality of our towns and cities. In other words, meteoropathy would in fact be a form of electrohypersensitivity (EHS), but in this case triggered by natural atmospheric factors.

To recap what has been explained so far, we know that cold fronts are especially associated with severe storms and are therefore strong generators of *sferics* (Vaitl *et al.*, 2001). Several independent research teams have demonstrated that *sferics* can induce headaches and changes in the electroencephalogram (EEG) (Shiencle *et al.*, 2001; Walach *et al.*, 2001). It is therefore to be expected that cold fronts show a stronger correlation with health symptoms and meteoropathy through the biophysical mechanisms described in our work (Panagopoulos and Balmori, 2017)—namely, ionic changes between the interior and exterior of cells caused by *sferics* through the activation or inhibition of ion channels in the cell membranes. As noted in Chapter 2, this is precisely what Taiwanese researchers have confirmed (without reference to *sferics*), documenting a close relationship between cold fronts and headaches (Yang *et al.*, 2011).

Consequently, the previously unknown reason why many people experience headaches and other symptoms during weather changes may finally be explained. By linking together the various published studies, we can conclude that *sferics*—particularly those associated with cold fronts—provoke headaches, EEG alterations, and other symptoms. This is what we shall attempt to demonstrate empirically in Chapter 4.

3.4 Unforeseen Effects

Several research teams have reported an increase in aggressiveness associated with atmospheric changes and have linked accident rates to the passage of weather fronts (Le Beau and Corcoran, 1990). Other authors have also connected criminal activity (Butke and Sheridan, 2010) and peaks in domestic violence (Auliciems and Di Bartolo, 1995) with meteorological conditions.

These correlations identified by different researchers are likely due to increased irritability associated with weather changes and the arrival of *sferics*, as suggested by Cherry (2002). This researcher proposed that the reduction in melatonin production caused by electromagnetic signals generally induces a rise in serotonin, which is associated with wakefulness, alertness, anxiety, anger, and violence—depending on an individual's temperament and circumstances.

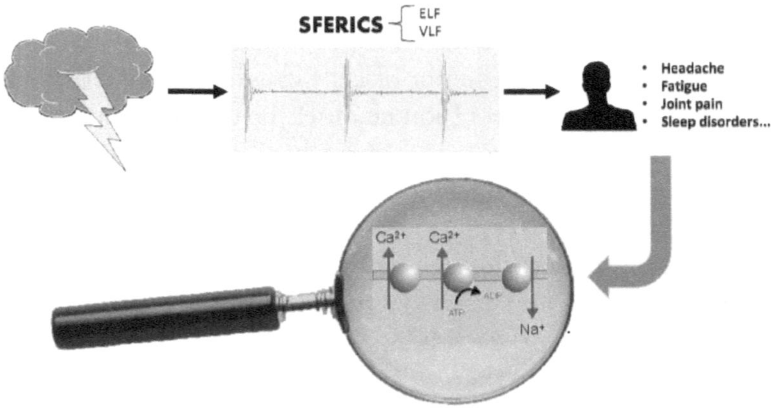

Figure 7. Sferics, generated by lightning particularly linked to cold fronts, disrupt the electrochemical balance and function of cell membranes, leading to headaches and other symptoms.

As a consequence of their effects on human health, wellbeing, and aggressiveness, *sferics* may have significant socio-economic repercussions. Indeed, daily work performance has also been found to correlate with daytime *sferic* activity (Warnke, 2007). For all these reasons, it remains both concerning and surprising that, knowing how sensitive we are to subtle natural radiations, we continue to saturate the very environments in which we live and work with countless and powerful artificial sources of electromagnetic radiation—such as those associated with new wireless information transmission systems and mobile telephony (see Chapter 5).

4

HEADACHES AND WEATHER MAPS

As mentioned in the previous chapter, several pioneering authors have suggested that *sferics* could be responsible for numerous meteoropathic conditions traditionally attributed—and still linked today—to conventional atmospheric parameters such as pressure, temperature, humidity, or solar radiation. We have also observed that, as sudden weather changes approach—particularly cold fronts—the appearance of *sferics* coincides temporally with the onset of symptoms associated with these conditions.

In this chapter, we shall take a step further and explore the possibility of linking a type of discomfort characteristic of weather-sensitive individuals—namely, headache or cephalalgia—with weather maps. To this end, we selected three people known to be particularly sensitive to weather changes and monitored their headache episodes over a five-year period, from October 2013 to November 2018. Following data collection (the recording of the dates on which headaches occurred), the corresponding meteorological maps were reviewed and analysed. The results obtained are presented in the following sections.

4.1 Coincidences in Different Individuals

Below are some of the atmospheric situations (weather maps or surface pressure charts), reviewed retrospectively, that were most frequently associated with headache episodes in the individuals studied. The meteorological data presented here were obtained from de Wetterzentrale [1], whose website provides the official daily weather records for Europe (with their explicit consent) over the past twenty years.

To rule out other possible headache triggers—such as stress, poor diet, or illness—only those episodes were selected in which all three participants experienced headaches simultaneously or on consecutive days.

First, we examine a case in which all three subjects experienced headaches at the same time. On 7 October 2013, two consecutive cold fronts approached from the Atlantic. On 8 October, all three individuals reported having headaches. By 9 October, the headaches had subsided, as the cold front moved inland across France (Map 1).

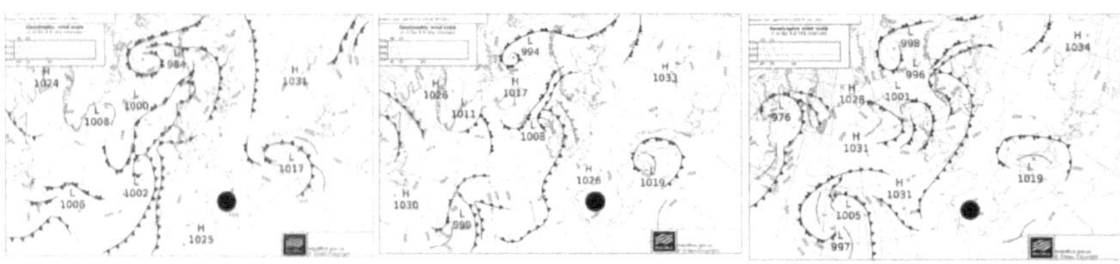

Map 1. Surface pressure charts for 7, 8, and 9 October 2013. The black dot indicates the approximate location of the individuals studied (Valladolid, Spain).

Next, four different episodes are examined in which all three individuals experienced headaches on consecutive days.

1 http://www.wetterzentrale.de/

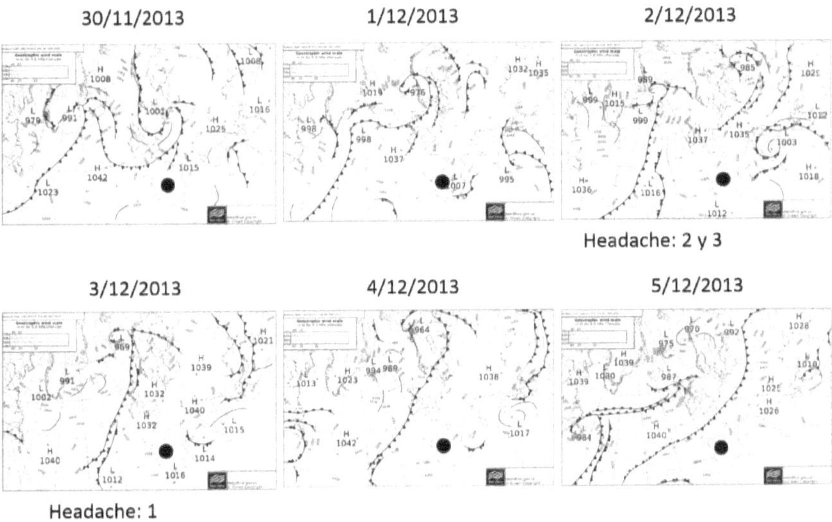

Map 2. Surface pressure charts for the indicated dates. On 2 December 2013, individuals 2 and 3 experienced headaches. The following day, individual 1 reported a headache. On 4 and 5 December, none of the three had headaches. The charts show that, during this period, a cold front approached from the Atlantic before subsequently veering northwards.

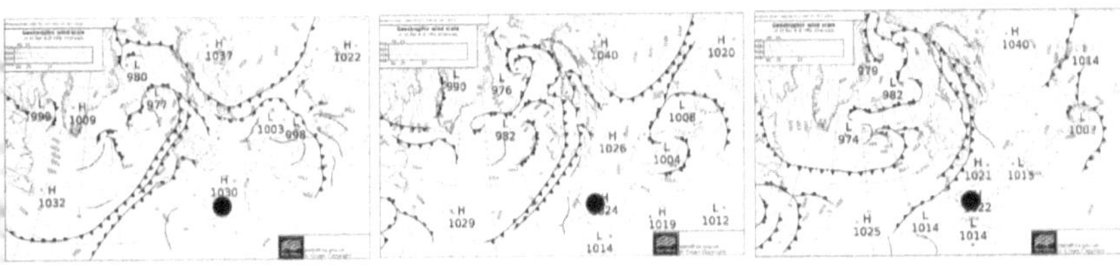

Map 3. Situation on 23, 24, and 25 October 2014. On 23 October, as many as three cold fronts approached from the Atlantic. On the 24th, there were two cold fronts, but closer to the peninsula. On the 25th, the cold front passed over and moved away from the peninsula. The three individuals experienced headaches on consecutive days: on 23 October, individuals 2 and 3 were affected; on the 24th, individual 1; and on the 25th, none of the three had headaches.

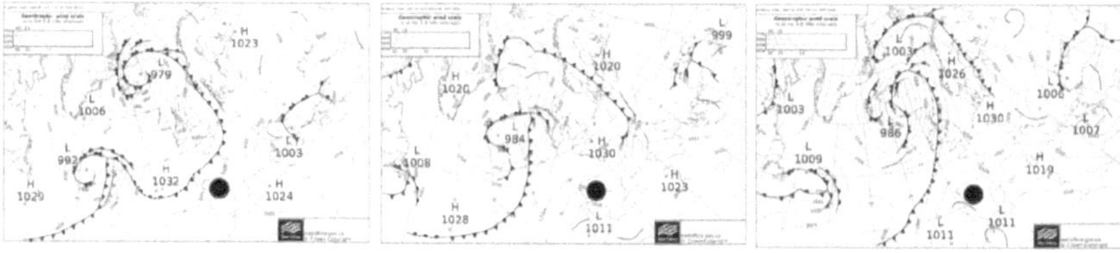

Map 4. Surface pressure charts for 3–5 May 2016. On 3 May, individual 3 experienced a headache; on the 4th, individual 2; and on the 5th, individual 1 — on consecutive days.

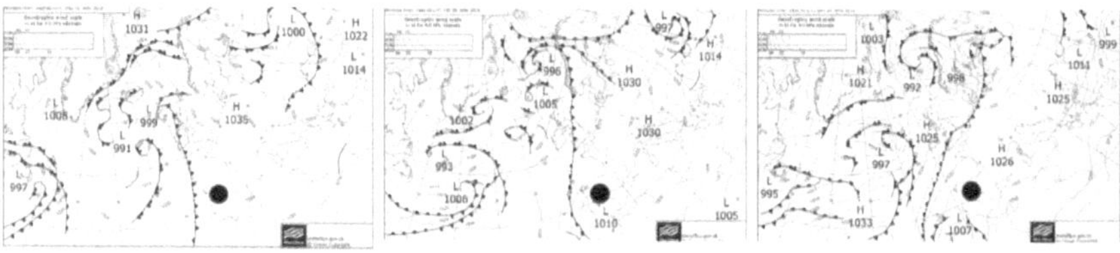

Map 5. Two consecutive cold fronts approached from the Atlantic between 19 and 21 April 2018. The three individuals studied experienced headaches on consecutive days: on 19 April, individual 2; on the 20th, individual 3; and on the 21st, individual 1.

The experience gained over the five-year observation period suggests that headache episodes tend to coincide with the approach of one or more cold fronts from the Atlantic. In the cases where all three individuals experienced headaches on consecutive days, it can be observed that individual 1 very often developed a headache one day after individuals 2 and 3. This pattern was repeated time and again throughout the period analysed, always occurring in the same order.

It should be emphasised that, on several dozen occasions, two of the three individuals experienced headaches either simultaneously or on consecutive days. However, the large number of such cases makes it impractical to describe them all in detail. Based on the experience accumulated over these years, the following seven typical meteorological situations are presented, each involving several consecutive cold fronts approaching from the Atlantic. These may cause headaches and other symptoms in weather-sensitive individuals, preceding the arrival of the depression over the Iberian Peninsula (Maps 6–12).

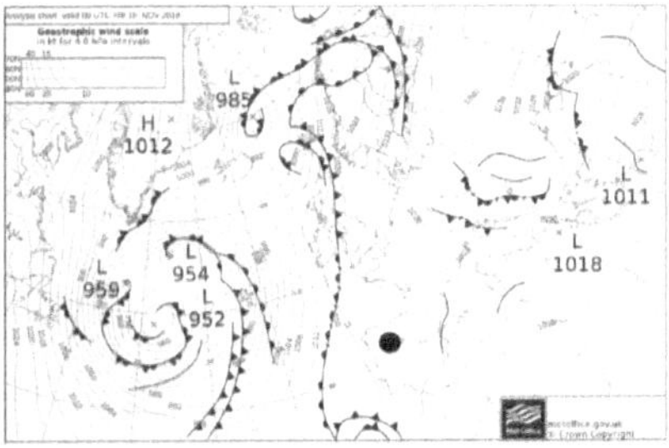

Map 6

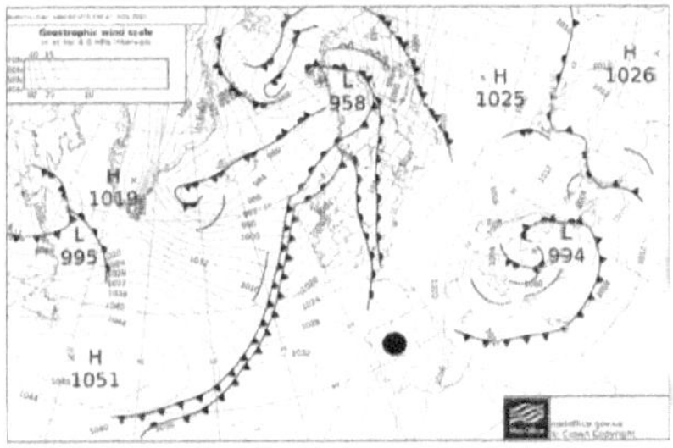

Map 7

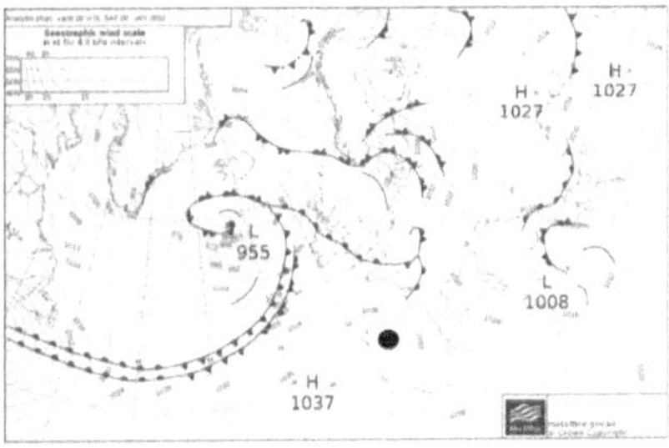

Map 8

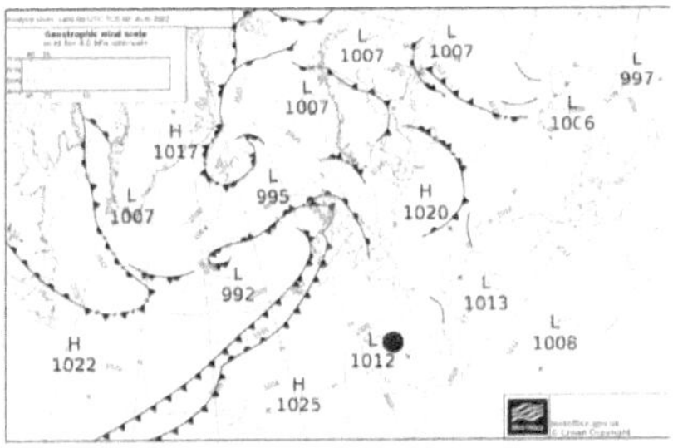

Map 9

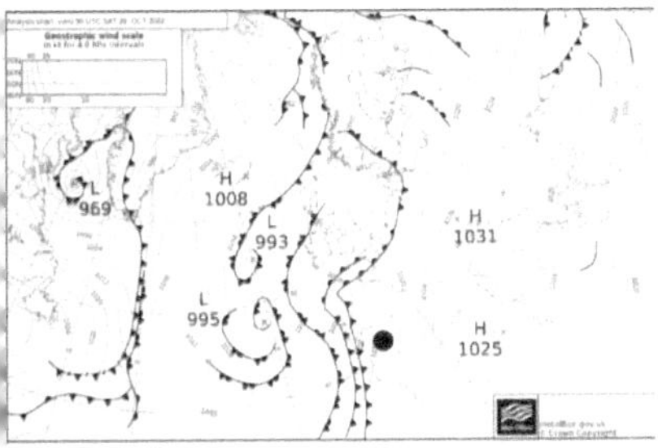

Map 10

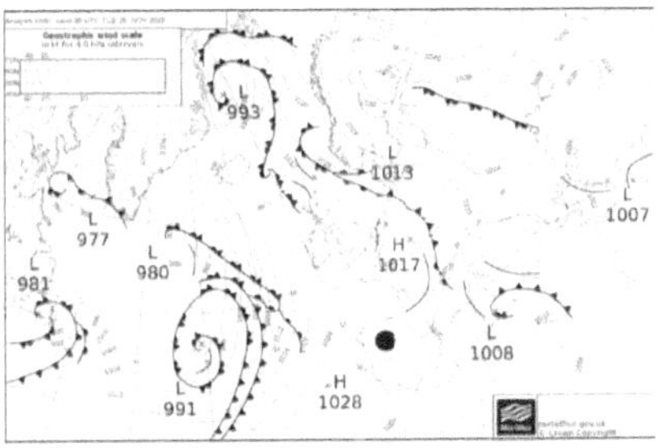

Map 11

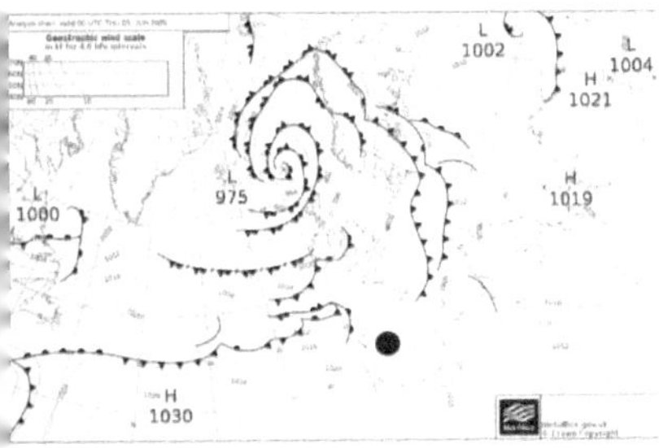

Map 12

4.2 General Conclusions of the Analysis

The results obtained during the follow-up of these three individuals confirm that headache episodes tend to occur between one and three days before the arrival of a cold front, when it is still located over the Atlantic Ocean at an approximate distance of between 2,000 and 1,000 kilometres. The onset of pain usually takes place during the night, often continuing into the following day and, in some cases, lasting for several consecutive days. These episodes would therefore appear to be related to the arrival of *sferics* generated by electrical discharges (lightning) in cold fronts over the Atlantic that are moving towards the Iberian Peninsula.

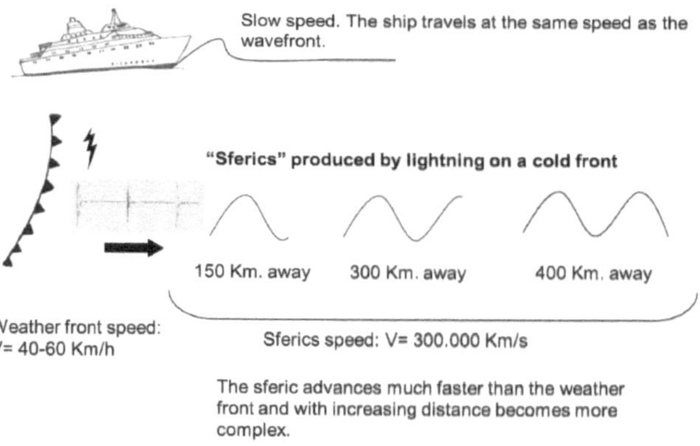

Figure 8. Comparison between the speed of a frontal wave generated by a ship and the speed of light at which sferics from electrical discharges associated with a cold front propagate.

Based on these findings, it is proposed that predictive weather maps could be used to anticipate, to some extent, the onset of headaches or other meteoropathic symptoms in individuals sensitive to weather changes. This predictive capability could have a significant impact both in the healthcare field and in the economic sphere. Conversely, the appearance of certain symptoms in weather-sensitive individuals could also serve as an early indicator of changing weather conditions, allowing the approach of cold fronts towards the Iberian Peninsula to be foreseen. This predictive ability would be linked to the arrival of *sferics*, since—unlike conventional meteorological factors such as pressure, temperature, or humidity, which only manifest with the arrival of the front or air mass—*sferics* travel at the speed of light and can be detected beforehand (Figure 8)..

4.3 New Questions and Some Possible Answers

During the course of investigating a new problem, it is common for unexpected questions to arise even as some of the initially posed issues begin to be resolved. This phenomenon highlights the unpredictable and deeply interwoven complexity of natural phenomena, particularly those concerning living beings and the natural world.

Could there be unknown physical reasons that account for some of the observations and questions raised? Fortunately, within the framework of current scientific knowledge, there are already some answers to these questions.

4.3.1 Why Does Headache (or Other Symptoms) Tend to Begin Especially at Night?

The propagation of *sferics* is more efficient during the night and over the ocean. Several studies attribute the reactions that occur while we sleep to the radiation of extremely low frequency (ELF) and very low frequency (VLF) electromagnetic waves, which are characteristic of the nocturnal period. It has been observed that the frequency of VLF emissions generated by lightning discharges shows a peak around midnight (Asada *et al.*, 2001).

This phenomenon is due to the changes that occur at night in the conditions of the waveguide —the region between the Earth's surface and the ionosphere— which enhance the transmission of *sferics* (Schienle *et al.*, 2001). Specifically, during the nighttime hours, the absence of solar radiation in the unilluminated hemisphere prevents ionisation of the ionosphere. Under these conditions, the propagation of *sferics* improves significantly — they can be transmitted up to a hundred times more efficiently than during the day (Warnke, 2007). The same effect has also been observed during solar eclipses, when darkness sets in suddenly. Measurements taken at specific receiving stations (Figure 9) confirm that the optimal conditions for the propagation of *sferics* occur over the ocean and during the night (Pessi *et al.*, 2009).

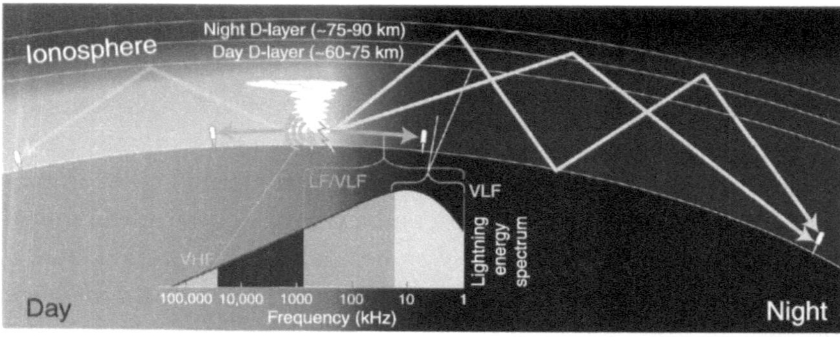

Figure 9. Schematic diagram of the waveguide formed between the Earth's surface and the ionosphere, which enables very low frequency (VLF, 3–30 kHz) emissions from thunderstorms (sferics) to propagate over thousands of kilometres through successive reflections. The most efficient propagation occurs over the ocean at night (right-hand side of the figure). Image reproduced from Pessi et al. (2009), with the authors' explicit permission.

All the cited publications provide convincing explanations for our observation — that headaches tend to begin more frequently at night — particularly when a cold front approaches over the sea, as generally happens in the Iberian Peninsula, where fronts typically move in from the west, originating over the Atlantic Ocean.

4.3.2 Why Do Some Weather Fronts Trigger Symptoms Sooner Than Others?

Cold fronts typically move at speeds of around 40 to 60 km/h. For instance, a front located 2,000 kilometres away and travelling at 40 km/h would take roughly 50 hours to arrive — about two days. If it were 1,000 kilometres away and maintained the same speed, its arrival would occur after about 25 hours (around one day). In contrast, if a front 2,000 kilometres distant were advancing at 60 km/h, it would reach its destination in approximately 33 hours. However, in all these cases, *sferics* arrive virtually instantaneously, as they propagate at the speed of light (Figure 8). For this reason, they can act as early indicators of meteorological changes, offering a predictive margin of between one and three days, depending on both the distance of the front and its rate of movement.

Since the speed of advance of cold fronts varies, this factor may partly explain the variability in the time interval between the perception and manifestation of meteoropathic symptoms. As observed in our analysis, meteorological fronts tend to be perceived at distances of between 1,000 and 2,000 kilometres — that is, roughly 24 to 48 hours before their arrival.

Moreover, this perception does not depend solely on external factors; individual variables also play a role, such as personal susceptibility, health status, and resilience capacity, all of which influence both the precise timing of symptom onset and their intensity.

4.3.3 Why Do Headaches Occur at a Specific Distance from the Front?

From the lightning generated in a storm, each of the resulting electromagnetic pulses — or *sferics* — becomes progressively more complex and loses intensity, that is, its amplitude diminishes, as it moves away from its point of origin (Figure 8). From an observation point located about 150–200 kilometres away, the *sferics* already display a complete sinusoidal oscillation. At a distance of around 300 kilometres, they take the form of a triple half-wave, and after travelling approximately 400 kilometres, the pulses exhibit a double-wave structure, with two full sinusoidal oscillations (Figures 8 and 10).

From this point onwards, their biotropic or bioactive potential — that is, their capacity to interact with biological systems — is considered to increase significantly. This is because the signal contains essential biochemical information: the sequence or frequency of the intervals between pulses. Such information may induce resonance phenomena and interfere with any biological or biochemical substrate that is sensitive or susceptible (Bäumer and Sönning, 2002).

Moreover, as discussed in Chapter 4, simultaneous atmospheric discharges of similar characteristics can produce transient constructive phenomena (interferences or couplings; Figure 5). In those locations, living organisms may be momentarily exposed to field intensities higher than those produced by single discharges (Panagopoulos and Balmori, 2017).

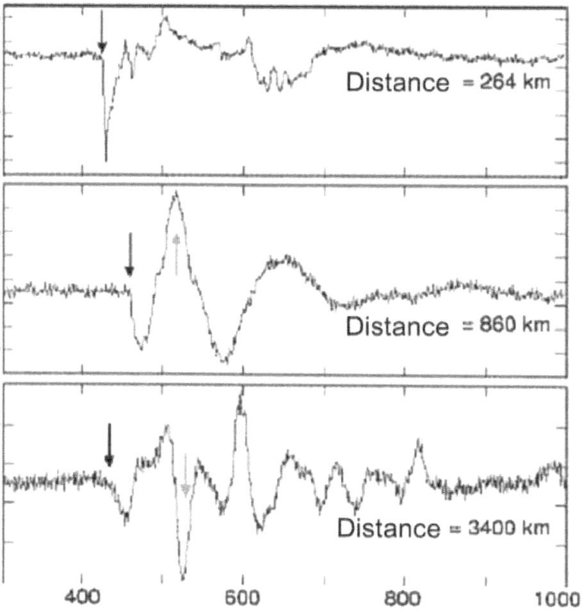

Figure 10.
(a)–(c) Vertical electric field waveforms for three cloud-to-ground lightning discharges detected by sensors located 264, 860, and 3,400 kilometres from the strike. The black arrow indicates the initial appearance of the wave at ground level. The grey arrows mark the first and second reflected waves. The horizontal axis represents elapsed time in microseconds. Image reproduced from Pessi et al. (2009), with the authors' explicit permission.

The period of time during which these biotropic waves reach us corresponds to when the symptoms appear. However, when the front gets too close (less than 500–1,000 kilometres away), its biotropic effects diminish, as there are no longer any reflected waves producing bioactive pulses. Lightning from nearby storms usually does not trigger such effects in the human body. In these cases — due to the storm's close proximity — the *sferics* are simple waves and do not yet contain low-frequency pulses capable of inducing resonance effects in the organism or interacting with biological systems (Figure 9). Nevertheless, some people are deeply afraid of thunderstorms, though this is more often associated with the deafening noise and fear of lightning strikes, frequently linked to unpleasant childhood experiences.

The perception of weather changes (such as the approach of weather fronts) is not exclusive to humans. The anecdotal observations mentioned earlier — spiders leaving their hiding places, sheep becoming more restless, and so on — suggest that *sferics* also produce similar effects in animals, prior to the arrival of weather fronts. This influence of electromagnetic pulses may also help explain the early-warning ability through which animals appear to sense earthquakes in advance (see Chapter 8).

4.3.4 Why Is There an Individual Difference in the Timing of Symptom Onset?

Figure 10 may help explain the individual differences in the perception of *sferics* and the onset of the associated symptoms. This is because the waveform changes with distance travelled, and each person may be sensitive to a specific type of waveform or pulse configuration. Depending on their individual characteristics — and possibly their genetic information — a person might respond more sensitively to a particular frequency or pulse pattern, anticipating the arrival of a cold front by one, two, or even three days (see Pessi *et al.*, 2009).

This could account for the individual differences observed in the perception of *sferics* — whether more distant or closer — and consequently in the early detection of weather changes. For instance, if Subject 3 experiences a headache a day earlier than Subject 1, this difference tends to repeat consistently with the arrival of each new front or meteorological change, as confirmed by the empirical analysis conducted. The person who perceives symptoms earlier generally does so consistently in each episode, suggesting that each individual is sensitive to a specific waveform or wave type associated with a particular distance travelled from its point of origin.

The width of the Atlantic Ocean ranges approximately from 2,800 km (between Brazil and Liberia) to 4,800 km (between the United States and Morocco). A front moving at an average speed of 50 km/h can cover about 3,600 km in three days. However, during this time the conditions of the front are likely to change, so under normal circumstances, the advance perception of its arrival rarely exceeds that three-day margin.

Finally, it is important to note that not all cold fronts located over the Atlantic actually reach the Iberian Peninsula, as they may deviate in other directions. In such cases, the typical premonitory symptoms of their approach may still be perceived, even though rainfall does not ultimately occur.

> *The author would appreciate receiving information from other individuals who are sensitive to weather changes and about how their experiences relate to the corresponding meteorological maps, in order to continue advancing in the understanding of this complex phenomenon. For this purpose, the following email address has been created: sfericsalfonso@gmail.com*
>
> *This is a citizen science initiative, in which everyone is invited to collaborate by contributing their own observations to help expand our knowledge. Comments of particular interest, considered especially relevant, may be included in future editions of this book, provided that the contributor gives their consent.*

5

THE UNCOMFORTABLE HYPOTHESIS

Technological radiation of human origin shares certain characteristics with natural *sferics*. In this chapter, we will see how, according to the existing scientific literature, various ailments and health problems have been reported among people living near mobile phone base stations (telecommunication antennas), similar to those previously associated with *sferics*. These symptoms have been grouped under the general term "microwave syndrome" or "radiofrequency sickness" (Gómez-Perretta *et al.*, 2013), more commonly known today as "electromagnetic hypersensitivity" (EHS). Both mobile phone antennas and handsets emit radiofrequency (RF) radiation, pulsed at extremely low frequencies (ELF), exposing humans to electric field intensities comparable to or even greater than those of natural *sferics* (Panagopoulos & Balmori, 2017).

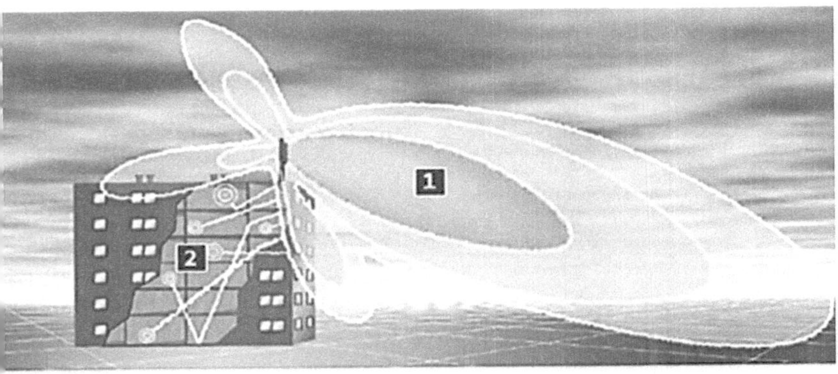

Figure 11: Typical radiation lobes from a mobile phone antenna located on the roof of a building.

5.1 Physical and Technological Characteristics of Mobile Telephony

Electromagnetic radiation transmits tiny packets of energy known as photons. Radiofrequencies occupy the range between 10 MHz and 300 GHz. Mobile phone base station antennas emit electromagnetic waves with a carrier frequency that depends on the generation of the system (for example, around 900 MHz for analogue systems, and 900 MHz and 1800 MHz for digital systems—see table). These are generally referred to as microwaves (approximately within the 1 GHz to 300 GHz range), pulsed at low frequencies. Microwaves convey sound information through short bursts or pulses with slight frequency modulations, which are exchanged between mobile phones and base stations.

Generation	Start Year	Key Technology	Frequency Band	Approximate Speed	Main Features
1G	1980s	Analogue (AMPS)	800 - 900 MHz	Up to 2.4 kbps	Voice only, low quality, no security
2G	1990s	Digital (GSM, CDMA)	850 MHz, 900 MHz, 1800 MHz, 1900 MHz	Up to 64 kbps	Digital voice, SMS, MMS, improved security
3G	2000s	UMTS, HSPA	850 MHz, 900 MHz, 1900 MHz, 2100 MHz	384 kbps several Mbps	Mobile internet, video calls, web browsing
4G	2010s	LTE	700 - 2600 MHz	10–100 Mbps (teórico Gbps)	*Streaming*, apps en tiempo real, juegos *online*
5G	From 2020	mmWave, sub-6 GHz	Sub-6 GHz: 600 MHz - 6 GHz mmWave: 24 GHz - 100 GHz	Up to 10 Gbps (theoretical)	Baja latencia, IoT, vehículos autónomos, ciudades inteligentes

The antenna of a mobile phone radiates in all directions through space, whereas the antenna of a base station produces a directional emission in the form of a lobe. In addition, several secondary lobes of lower power are generated, extending sideways and to the rear in the vicinity of the antenna. Mobile phone base stations usually consist of three sectors, each equipped with an antenna covering an angle of 120 degrees, which together provide full 360-degree coverage.

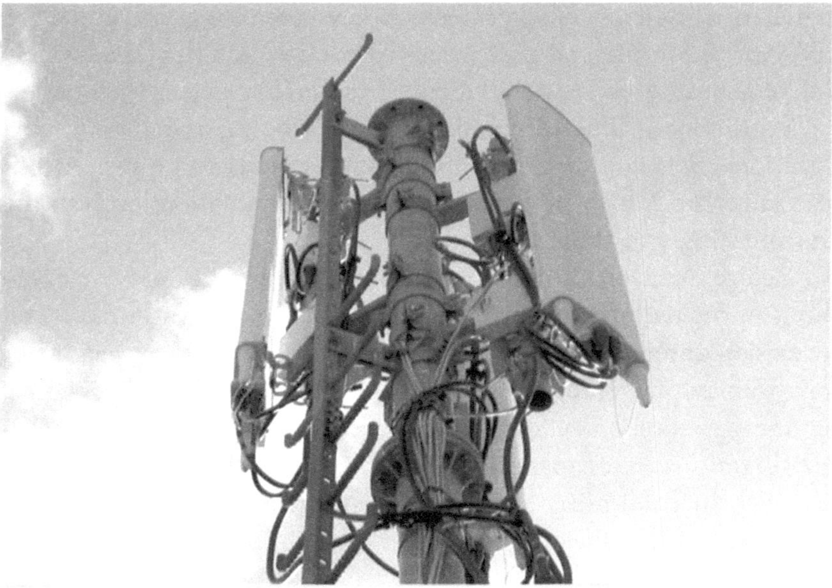

Figure 12: Close-up of a mobile phone base station typically oriented in three spatial directions, each antenna covering an angle of 120°..

One of the main units used to measure this type of radiation is power density (measured in watts per square metre: W/m², or in microwatts per square centimetre: μW/cm²), which expresses the radiant power incident perpendicularly on a surface, divided by the surface area. Another commonly used quantity is the electric field strength at a given point (measured in volts per metre: V/m), a vector quantity proportional to the force exerted on a charged particle, and dependent on its position in space.

In a specific direction relative to the antenna, power density decreases with the square of the distance from the emitting source, assuming propagation takes place in free space without obstacles, reflections or additional attenuation. At a distance of 50 metres from a mobile phone antenna, the typical power density is around 10 $\mu W/cm^2$ (6.1 V/m), while at distances of 100 metres at ground level it can still measure above 1 $\mu W/cm^2$ (2 V/m). Between 150 and 200 metres, the power density of the main lobe near the ground is on the order of tenths of a $\mu W/cm^2$. Biological effects have been suggested above 0.1 $\mu W/cm^2$ (0.6 V/m), and power density levels exceed this value widely in areas located less than 300 metres from mobile phone antennas.

Furthermore, due to the difficulty of finding suitably elevated locations, it is common for several base stations to be installed at the same site, which proportionally increases radiation levels in the surrounding area (Figure 16).

Before the deployment of wireless telephony, existing wave emissions in the radiofrequency range originated mainly from radio and television antennas, which were usually installed at great heights or far from populated areas. Since the 1990s, the roll-out of mobile phone base station networks has increased electromagnetic pollution by several orders of magnitude, especially in urban environments, but also in rural areas and near transport infrastructures such as motorways and railway lines.

5.2 The Effects of Technological Radiation on Human Beings

Professor Neil Cherry, a researcher at Lincoln University in New Zealand, who passed away in 2003, carried out an immense amount of work warning of the health impacts associated with the development of new wireless technologies. Dr Cherry came from a background in meteorology and was particularly interested in biometeorology.

He devoted much of his research and scientific reviews to demonstrating the non-thermal effects of electromagnetic radiation on cancer, memory, aggression, the release of melatonin by the pineal gland, genotoxic effects (those that damage DNA), as well as impacts on the circulatory and reproductive systems, and on neurodegenerative diseases—one of which eventually confined him to a wheelchair during his final years and led to his premature death. His early warnings have been increasingly confirmed over time, as a substantial body of subsequent scientific studies has fully supported his pioneering concerns.

Another researcher who was also an early voice warning about the possible risks of wireless telephony—though likewise largely ignored—was the British biophysicist G. L. Hyland of the University of Warwick. In 2000, Hyland published an article in the renowned medical journal *The Lancet*, entitled "Physics and biology of mobile telephony" (Hyland, 2000). In that paper, he explained how, although mobile phone safety standards, along with those for base stations and other wireless technologies, protect against excessive heating, there is evidence that low-intensity pulsed radiation may exert subtle non-thermal influences. He suggested that if such influences were found to have adverse health consequences, current safety limits would be inadequate.

Dr Hyland further remarked that the oscillatory similarity between pulsed microwave radiation and certain electrochemical activities within the human body should be a cause for concern—though he made clear that not all individuals would be affected in the same way. He emphasised the importance of the fact that these waves are pulsed, a property which, as we have also seen in the case of *sferics*, characterises their biotropic or biological activity. Hyland explained that the human body is an exquisitely sensitive electrochemical instrument whose orderly functioning and regulation depend on oscillatory electrical processes of various kinds, each characterised by a specific frequency—and that some of these frequencies are very close to those used in mobile telephony. For this reason, certain electrical activities within the body may be interfered with by the oscillatory properties of the incident radiation, in much the same way that electromagnetic waves cause interference in radio receivers (as we have also seen with atmospheric *sferics*, which produce similar effects).

Thus, unlike thermal effects—which depend on the body's ability to absorb energy from the electromagnetic field—the possibility of non-thermal effects arises from an oscillatory similarity between the radiation and the living organism. This makes it possible for the organism to respond to low-intensity pulsed radiation through its capacity to recognise certain features of that radiation (such as frequency, pulses, and modulation).

Dr Hyland provided a clear example of human vulnerability to a non-thermal effect of electromagnetic radiation: the capacity of a flashing light, flickering at a frequency of approximately 15 Hz (15 pulses per second), to induce seizures in people with photosensitive epilepsy. In this case, it is not the amount of energy emitted by the light (its intensity) that triggers the seizure, but rather the information conveyed to the brain by the regularity (coherence) of the flicker, at a frequency that the brain particularly "recognises". This "recognition" occurs because the pulse frequency coincides with or approximates that used by the brain itself (Hyland, 2000), and it can also affect brain waves (EEG), just as natural pulsed radiation from atmospheric discharges (*sferics*) can.

As with *sferics*, there are numerous reports of headaches in mobile phone users (Chu *et al.*, 2011). One possible explanation that has been suggested for these headaches relates to the characteristics of the electromagnetic fields emitted by mobile phones, which may increase the permeability of the blood–brain barrier and allow harmful substances to enter the brain, thereby damaging neurons (Salford *et al.*, 2003).

Professor Hyland, deeply concerned by the rapid deployment of mobile telephony at the beginning of the twenty-first century without an adequate evaluation of its effects on living organisms, warned about this situation—one that has continued unabated to the present day. For this reason, he produced a report for the European Parliament entitled "The physiological and environmental effects of non-ionising electromagnetic radiation" (Hyland, 2001). In that report, he warned that one of the main threats to public health is *electropollution* (also known as *electrosmog*) generated by human activity.

This non-ionising electromagnetic pollution of technological origin is particularly insidious because it escapes human sensory perception—something that tends to encourage an unconscious attitude towards both its use and personal protection. Furthermore, human beings have no defences against potential interference with the natural electromagnetic processes upon which our homeostasis—or internal balance—depends, such as the Schumann resonance. As discussed in Chapter 3, this resonance consists of a weak electromagnetic field oscillating resonantly in the space between the Earth's surface and the ionosphere, at frequencies close to those of the human brain. It has been found that isolation from this natural radiation harms health (Hyland, 2000).

In 2010, Americans B. Levitt and H. Lai from the University of Washington published an important review in the journal *Environmental Reviews* on the biological effects of exposure to electromagnetic radiation emitted by mobile phone base stations. Their aim was to review studies conducted on people living or working near such infrastructures, who are therefore chronically exposed to low-level radiofrequency radiation. Like Dr Hyland, these authors also warned that electromagnetic fields are among the fastest-growing forms of environmental pollution. Both anecdotal observations and epidemiological studies have reported headaches, skin rashes, sleep disturbances, depression, reduced libido, increased suicide rates, concentration and memory problems, dizziness, increased cancer risk, tremors, and other neurophysiological effects among populations living near base stations (note the similarities with the effects of *sferics*—natural pulsed radiations with similar physical characteristics—described in previous chapters).

One of the most interesting findings emerging from studies of populations exposed to radiation from mobile phone antennas is an increase in irritability (Johnson, 1998; Santini *et al.*, 2003; Abdel-Rassoul *et al.*, 2007; Eger and Jahn, 2010; Khurana *et al.*, 2010; Levitt and Lai, 2010; Gómez-Perretta *et al.*, 2013; Shahbazi-Gahrouei *et al.*, 2014)—a reaction also observed in response to the approach of weather fronts.

The widespread use of mobile telephony began during the 1990s. Since then, debate about the alleged effects of this technology on human health and the environment has never ceased—and indeed appears to have grown more intense in recent years. To an observer unacquainted with the complexity of the issue, it may appear that the "scientific world" is polarised between two opposing positions: on the one hand, those who claim that the levels recommended by the ICNIRP (International Commission on Non-Ionizing Radiation Protection) are sufficient to safeguard human health and the environment (see Chapter 7); and on the other, those who argue that these levels must be drastically reduced, since current recommendations fail to take into account the non-thermal effects on living organisms and the cumulative effects of continuous exposure to low-intensity radiation.

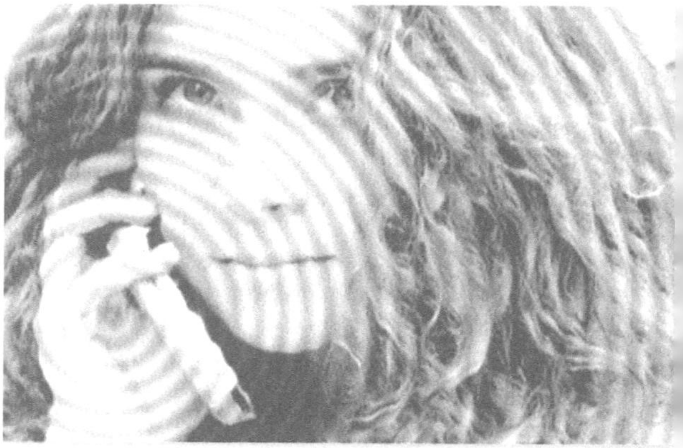

Figure 13: All living beings—and especially humans—are exposed to electromagnetic radiation of technological origin.

Over the past twenty years, hundreds of studies have been published and major scientific advances have taken place, tipping the balance towards those scientists calling for caution and for a reduction in the levels of exposure to which living beings are subjected. Epidemiological studies conducted with mobile phone users indicate that prolonged use may lead to long-term effects such as ocular problems (Dovrat *et al.*, 2005), hearing impairment (García Callejo *et al.*, 2005), alterations in the blood–brain barrier (Salford *et al.*, 2003), and reproductive issues (Davoudi *et al.*, 2002).

In addition, studies carried out in the vicinity of mobile phone base stations have revealed health problems—commonly referred to as the microwave syndrome or electrohypersensitivity—among residents living near these installations (Hutter *et al.*, 2002; Santini *et al.*, 2003; Navarro *et al.*, 2003; Oberfeld *et al.*, 2004). In such epidemiological studies, cancer cases have been found to be up to four times higher in the areas closest to antennas (Eger *et al.*, 2004; Wolf and Wolf, 2004). Some plausible models of tumour promotion by these radiations have been proposed and have attracted considerable attention among specialists (Leszczynski *et al.*, 2002). According to these models, radiation from mobile phones is absorbed by brain tissue and activates stress proteins (hsp 27), increasing the permeability of the blood–brain barrier and altering the pattern of apoptosis (programmed cell death), thereby preventing the elimination of old or transformed cells (those that have sustained DNA damage).

Prior to the introduction of third-generation mobile technology (UMTS), the Dutch government commissioned a study which found cognitive and health alterations associated with exposure to emissions from UMTS mobile phone antennas (Zwamborn *et al.*, 2003).

5.3 Irrefutable Scientific Evidence

Over the past few decades, hundreds of thousands of mobile phone base stations and other types of wireless telecommunications antennas have been installed across the world, both in urban and rural areas—including protected natural zones—adding to the already existing infrastructure for television, broadcasting, radar, and so on. In general, the deployment of these systems has taken into account only aesthetic considerations or urban planning regulations. To date, however, no comprehensive assessment has been made of the biological, environmental, or health impacts of non-ionising electromagnetic radiation emissions. Consequently, neither the environmental degradation nor the potential health effects on people living or working in the vicinity of these antennas have been properly considered.

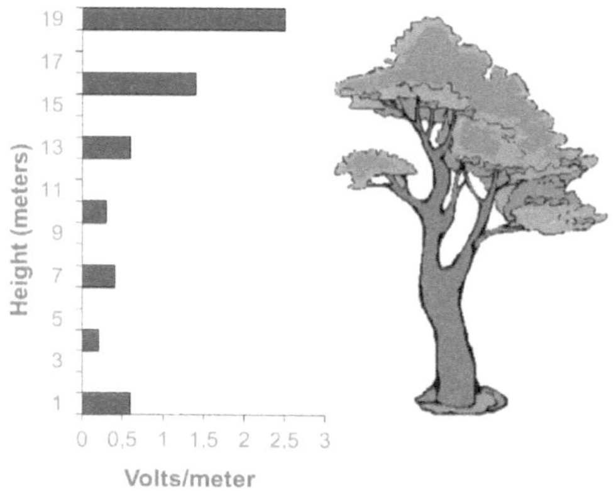

Figure 14:
Electric field intensity at different heights above ground level (actual data measured 100 metres from a base station). Note that the values increase with height as they enter the antenna's main emission lobe. For this reason, radiation tends to affect the upper parts of trees and the highest floors of residential buildings in particular. (Image from Balmori [2004], with measurements by the autor).

Estimates have shown that radiofrequency (RF) electromagnetic fields from mobile phone systems are stronger in urban areas than in rural ones. However, total exposure varies not only between urban and rural environments but also according to the specific characteristics of individual dwellings. For instance, in multi-storey buildings, higher levels of radiation exposure are generally observed on the upper floors (Breckenkamp *et al.*, 2012; see Figure 14).

As explained at the beginning of this chapter, there is a specific symptom pattern associated with exposure to low-intensity radiofrequencies, characterised by functional disturbances of the central nervous system—such as headaches, insomnia, discomfort, irritability, depression, memory loss, dizziness, fatigue, nausea, loss of appetite, and difficulty concentrating. This condition has been referred to as radiofrequency sickness (Lilienfeld *et al.*, 1978; Johnson Lyakouris, 1998; Navarro *et al.*, 2003).

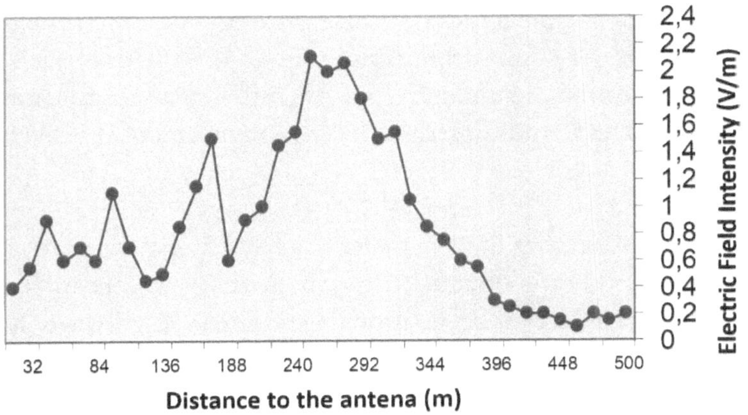

Figure 15: Variation in electric field intensity at ground level as a function of distance from a mobile phone base station located 24 metres above ground, on the rooftop of a building. In general, the highest levels of radiation are recorded at distances between 50 and 300 metres from the antenna (data from the author)..

In the summer of 2022, I published a review article in the prestigious scientific journal *Environmental Research*, with the eloquent title "Evidence of a health risk from radiofrequency radiation in humans living near mobile phone base stations: from radiofrequency sickness to cancer." The aim of that study was to conduct a comprehensive review of the available literature in order to update current knowledge on the possible health effects of mobile phone base stations on people living in their vicinity.

To this end, I examined all the scientific literature published on the effects of mobile phone base stations located near residential areas. The overall results revealed three main categories of health effects associated with base station antennas: radiofrequency sickness, cancer, and changes in biochemical parameters. Of the 38 studies analysed worldwide, 73.6% (28 out of 38) reported health effects: 73.9% (17 out of 23) in relation to radiofrequency sickness; 76.9% (10 out of 13) in cancer cases; and 75.0% (6 out of 8) regarding alterations in biochemical parameters.

Taken together, most of these investigations—carried out by research teams from twenty different countries—converge in their conclusions, providing a coherent picture of the health effects observed among people living near base stations. Moreover, the observation of similar effects from other sources of radiation, such as radar installations, radio and television antennas, wireless smart meters, and laboratory studies, reinforces the robustness of this overall assessment

5.3.1 Research Involving Radar and Radio/Television Antennas

A number of studies conducted throughout the past century have documented the effects of occupational exposure to microwave (RF) radiation associated with military and industrial applications, as well as to radio waves. Among the effects observed are an increased rate of spontaneous abortions, alterations in red and white blood cell counts, and a higher incidence of childhood cancer. These findings support the hypothesis that exposure to RF radiation may be potentially carcinogenic and entail other health risks.

Furthermore, analyses based on the specific localisation of diagnosed neoplasms indicate significantly higher morbidity rates among military personnel exposed to RF radiation, particularly in cancers of the digestive tract, skin tumours, and malignant neoplasms of cerebral and haematological/lymphatic origin.

In addition, a study conducted by Kolodynski and Kolodynska (1996) found that children exposed to electromagnetic radiation generated by radar installations showed reduced development of memory and attention, slower reaction times, and diminished neuromuscular endurance.

5.3.2 Havana Syndrome

Between late 2016 and August 2017, U.S. diplomatic personnel stationed in Havana, Cuba, reported a range of neurological symptoms, including cognitive, balance, visual, and auditory impairments, as well as sleep disturbances and headaches. These individuals exhibited signs of widespread brain network damage, despite having no history of traumatic brain injury. The most frequent symptoms included cognitive impairment, fatigue, and headaches, especially after mental exertion. In some cases, tinnitus, nausea, and balance problems were also reported.

This mysterious condition, which affected U.S. and Canadian diplomats in Cuba—and later in China as well—has baffled the FBI, the State Department, and various U.S. intelligence agencies. The collected reports suggest that the observed neurological lesions may be related to exposure to microwaves or pulsed radio frequencies (Golomb, 2018). In line with this hypothesis, a report from the U.S. National Academy of Sciences (2020) concluded that many of the reported chronic or nonspecific symptoms—such as dizziness, headache, fatigue, nausea, anxiety, cognitive impairment, and memory loss—are consistent with the known effects of radiofrequency exposure. Taken together, the evidence suggests that pulsed, specifically targeted radiofrequency energy is the most plausible mechanism to explain these cases. In fact, objective pathophysiological changes and detrimental health effects resulting from exposure to electromagnetic fields have been identified, which can cause biological damage in previously healthy individuals (Belpomme and Irigaray, 2022).

5.3.3 The Precautionary Principle

As will be discussed in greater depth in Chapter 7, the International Commission on Non-Ionizing Radiation Protection (ICNIRP) is a private organisation that sets guidelines for exposure levels to electromagnetic fields, which are adopted by many governments. However, this body has faced criticism for potential conflicts of interest. The exposure limits proposed by the ICNIRP are thousands of times higher than the levels at which biological effects associated with anthropogenic extremely low frequency (ELF) and radiofrequency (RF) electromagnetic fields have been documented. Moreover, these guidelines are based exclusively on thermal effects — that is, those involving a rise in tissue temperature — while disregarding the substantial scientific evidence concerning non-thermal effects. Current regulations only take into account the risks arising from acute, high-intensity exposures, offering no protection against chronic, low-intensity exposure. Yet, the duration of exposure is a key factor in assessing potential health effects.

The precautionary principle is one of the fundamental pillars of the European Union's approach to environmental protection, public health, and food safety (Harremoes *et al.*, 2013). This principle empowers policymakers to take preventive action even when the available scientific evidence about an environmental or health risk is inconclusive, provided that the possibility of harm cannot be ruled out with certainty. Nevertheless, despite the growing and consistent empirical evidence on the adverse effects of electromagnetic fields, no significant progress has been made by the competent authorities and regulatory bodies in updating official guidelines. Several authors have noted that study outcomes in this field often correlate with funding sources, and that many systematic reviews and meta-analyses have not adequately corrected for this bias — a factor that has likely contributed to an underestimation of the level of evidence regarding causality.

For this reason, as will be discussed later, an increasing number of scientists have urged governments and international organisations to review and strengthen safety standards for exposure to radiofrequency electromagnetic fields. Consequently, there is an urgent need to apply the precautionary principle effectively and to impose stricter exposure limits that adequately protect public health. A general principle holds that any potentially harmful agent should be properly assessed before being introduced to the public market. Mobile phones do not comply with this principle.

In the current situation, it is clear that scientists specialising in the study of electromagnetic field effects are fully aware of the seriousness of the issue, as demonstrated by the numerous scientific appeals made in recent years (see Chapter 7). However, this crucial information is not being effectively communicated to the public by the media, the relevant authorities — particularly the World Health Organization — or governments, thereby contributing to a widespread state of public misinformation.

As a result, this lack of adequate response is likely to lead not only to a public health crisis, but also to one concerning the very development and sustainability of this technology, which poses risks to both the environment and human wellbeing.

One of the consequences of recent scientific findings is that the European Recommendation 1999/519/EC — incorporated into Spanish legislation and based on ICNIRP exposure levels — has become outdated. Given the accumulated evidence, these limits should be urgently reviewed in order to ensure effective protection of public health.

5.4 The Silenced Reality

Another issue of particular importance, parallel to the use of mobile phones, concerns people's exposure to mobile phone masts located near their homes or workplaces for many hours each day — a kind of involuntary and unauthorised human experiment. The environment of these individuals is contaminated by a form of pollution that cannot be seen or directly perceived. This is a wholly unacceptable situation that raises serious ethical concerns. In other words, for all practical purposes, they are the involuntary subjects of a large-scale experiment (Hyland, 2001). The stubborn reality is that those who live or work in the vicinity of mobile phone base stations cannot decide for themselves the level of electromagnetic radiation to which they wish to be exposed.

Many estate agents know from direct experience — though often without fully understanding the underlying cause — that numerous top-floor flats and penthouses are difficult to rent or sell, change tenants frequently, and remain vacant for extended periods. When mobile phone antennas are visible from these properties and positioned at a similar height, these dwellings are often those receiving the highest direct exposure to radiation. This, in turn, contributes to the economic depreciation of the property, leaving owners powerless to act.

Children with persistent crying, parents suffering from insomnia, and individuals with unexplained symptoms that elude diagnosis through conventional medical examinations — which, regrettably, rarely investigate environmental causes or the everyday ecology of those affected — have led many families to abandon their homes or, at best, to attempt to protect themselves by installing metal sheets, using the well-known Faraday cage method. This is the reality that has been emerging for years, and it is well understood that, like science itself, the truth cannot remain hidden indefinitely.

Figura 16: Three mobile phone base stations on the roof of a hotel, affecting the health and sleep quality of residents living on the upper floors of nearby buildings, as well as the hotel's own guests.

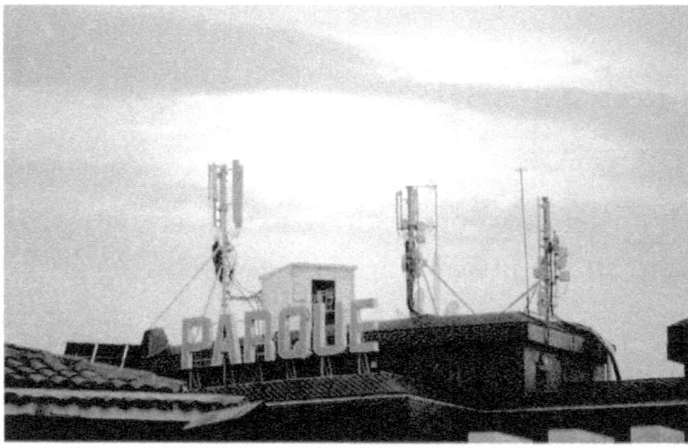

Mobile phone networks have expanded and been deployed at an unrestrained pace over the past twenty-five years, often at the expense of numerous urban planning and legal irregularities, both in Spain and in other countries. The chaotic and uncontrolled proliferation of antennas has resulted in a marked increase in electromagnetic pollution and in the associated environmental and health risks.

Although company spokespeople continually repeat in the media that "nothing has been proven" and often seek to ridicule those affected, radiofrequency illness — also referred to as microwave syndrome — is a recognised medical condition encompassing a range of common symptoms (headache, fatigue, irritability, loss of appetite, sleep disorders, depression, difficulty concentrating, memory loss, visual and auditory disturbances, vertigo, impaired motor coordination, and cardiovascular, dermatological and immunological problems, among others). These symptoms have been reported in epidemiological studies involving individuals living near mobile phone base stations. Their incidence increases significantly as the distance from the emitting source decreases (Santini *et al.*, 2003), and their severity correlates directly with the power density measured in each dwelling (Navarro *et al.*, 2003). It is important to recall that the radiation emitted by antennas and mobile phones is the same — modulated and pulsed microwaves. The implementation of UMTS and 5G systems requires multiplying the number of antennas, and it is foreseeable that this will further exacerbate electromagnetic pollution.

As discussed throughout this book, living organisms are highly sensitive electrochemical systems that interact with their environment through electrical impulses. Within our bodies, ionic currents and electrical potential differences exist across cell membranes and within intra- and extracellular fluids. The electromagnetic fields generated within biological structures are characterised by specific frequencies, which may be interfered with by incident electromagnetic radiation, inducing alterations and modifying biological responses.

The saturation of our surroundings with artificially generated electromagnetic emissions across a wide range of frequencies has negative consequences for living beings. For this reason, monitoring and control are essential. Certain organs and systems, such as the heart and the nervous system, are particularly sensitive to such inductions. For example, several studies have demonstrated that the low-frequency pulses used in the GSM system interfere with brain waves, inducing delta waves — which are pathological in awake adults. The European recommendation to exercise caution in the use of mobile phones by individuals with pacemakers stems from the same concern.

Robert O. Becker, the late pioneering researcher and author of *The Body Electric*, stated some years ago: “I have no doubt that, at present, the most serious pollutant in the Earth’s environment — even more serious than global climate change and chemical pollution — is the proliferation of electromagnetic radiation.”

Industry representatives often seek to convince the public that the power output of mobile phone antennas is similar to that of ordinary household appliances. What they fail to explain, however, is that the alternating current (50–60 Hz) in household devices, cables and transformers induces a static electromagnetic field that does not propagate through space, diminishes within a few decimetres of the source, and disappears once the power is switched off. In contrast, mobile phone antennas emit microwave radiation that travels outward from the source, persists even when the source is turned off, and can reach distances of many kilometres.

They are also misleading when they claim that the strongest electromagnetic pollution comes from broadcasting frequencies. In reality, the frequencies assigned to mobile telephony account for the majority of electromagnetic pollution in urban environments, which has risen exponentially in recent years.

At present, operators are attempting to overcome public resistance to the installation of antennas through new camouflage strategies. The placement of small "pico-antennas" at street level particularly affects pedestrians and shop premises, effectively contaminating entire streets (whereas rooftop antennas mainly affect residents of upper floors). Although the long-term outcome is still uncertain, alarming reports are emerging of significant increases in insomnia and neurodegenerative diseases among elderly people.

A common tactic when negotiating the installation of a new antenna on a rooftop is to threaten property owners that, should they refuse, it will simply be placed on the neighbouring building — claiming that this would be even more harmful to them. Another frequent strategy to divert attention is to emphasise the risks associated with ionising radiation while downplaying or denying those linked to non-ionising radiation. Nevertheless, low-frequency (50–60 Hz) non-ionising electromagnetic fields were classified in June 2001 as a "possible human carcinogen" (Group 2B) by the expert committee of the International Agency for Research on Cancer (IARC), responsible for the classification of carcinogenic agents.

Although politicians and the media often seek to "reassure" the public by claiming that electromagnetic radiation levels comply with current regulations, there is considerable disparity among the maximum public exposure limits set by different countries. In Spain, the legislation allows a maximum power density of up to 450 μW/cm² for GSM frequencies (900 MHz). However, countries such as Italy, Hungary, Poland and Luxembourg set limits roughly 45 times stricter, while Switzerland and the region of Wallonia (Belgium) apply regulations between 90 and 105 times more restrictive. In Russia, the permitted levels are up to 450 times lower than those in Spain. These differences reflect markedly divergent approaches to public health protection in relation to electromagnetic field exposure, and underscore the urgent need to review and harmonise safety standards to ensure adequate protection.

The refusal of insurance companies to assume liability for potential harm caused by this technology — despite the vast profits it generates — is particularly concerning. Equally striking is the complete absence of signed statements by professionals certifying the absolute safety of such radiation. As we have seen, operators tend to invoke compliance with regulations whose reliability is questionable and which contain evident contradictions, using ambiguous terms such as "sensitive areas", "safety limits", or "decision levels".

Nor is it often mentioned that the Specific Absorption Rate (SAR), used to indicate the level of radiation emitted by mobile phones, is based on a highly artificial and limited model. This measure was standardised using tests on an inanimate mannequin made of a homogeneous plastic mass filled with saline solution, designed to simulate the thermal conductivity of human tissue. However, this model entirely lacks the physiological, structural and reactive properties that characterise living organisms.

As a result, SAR values account only for immediate thermal effects of exposure, without considering non-thermal effects or potential harm arising from prolonged or repeated exposure over time. A useful analogy would be assessing the risk of alcohol addiction solely on the basis of whether daily consumption stays below a fixed threshold — while completely ignoring the cumulative effects of continued intake over months or years.

5.5 The Tragic Case of García Quintana School

Between 2000 and 2003, an unusual cluster of cancer cases with a clear spatial and temporal concentration was recorded at the García Quintana Public School in Valladolid. Six cases of cancer were documented, five of which involved children and one a cleaning staff member. The first case occurred in the year 2000 — a four-year-old girl diagnosed with leukaemia. In 2001, three new cases appeared: two boys aged nine and six, and a five-year-old girl. In November 2003, another lymphoma was diagnosed. Tragically, one of the affected children, Carla, aged seven, passed away. The sixth case, revealed in May 2004, corresponded to a lymphoma diagnosed in 2002 in a school employee. Some years later, the head teacher also died of leukaemia. All the cases were haematological in nature and occurred within the same classroom block, sharing a similar orientation.

A notable feature of the surrounding environment was the presence of a dense cluster of mobile phone antennas installed in the immediate vicinity of the school (see Figure 17). Although the exact number of antennas and their transmission power were never officially clarified, their proximity and direct alignment with the affected classrooms raised serious concern about potential exposure to radiofrequency electromagnetic fields (RF-EMF) as an environmental risk factor.

In response to public alarm and under pressure from the Parents' Association (AMPA), the Public Prosecutor's Office intervened, leading to a court order that required the antennas to be dismantled in December 2001. This action took place in the same year that the highest number of cases (three) had been recorded. Since that cluster, no new cancer cases have occurred at the school, reinforcing the hypothesis of a causal relationship between environmental exposure to electromagnetic radiation and the emergence of the cluster.

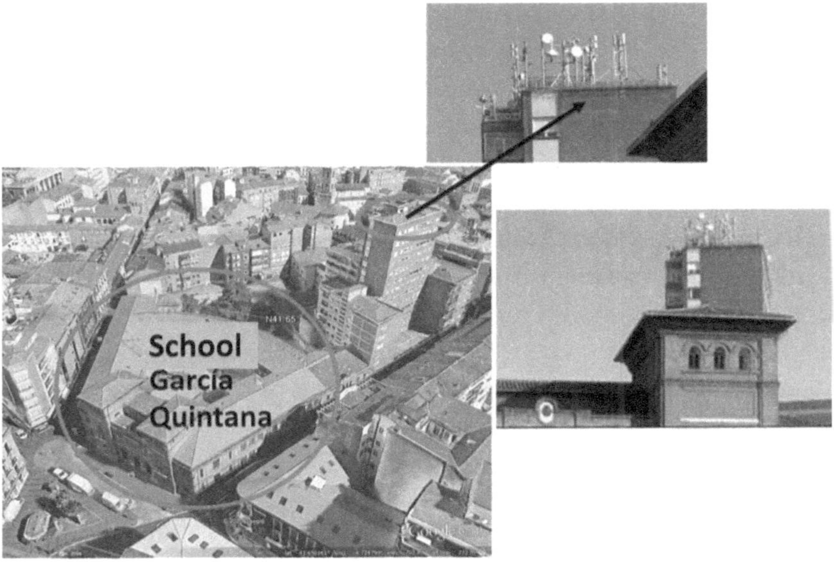

Figure 17. Diagram of the García Quintana Public School and the concentration of mobile phone antennas on an adjacent building.

In response to public alarm and under pressure from the Parents' Association (AMPA), the Public Prosecutor's Office intervened, leading to a court order that required the antennas to be dismantled in December 2001. This action took place in the same year that the highest number of cases (three) had been recorded. Since that cluster, no new cancer cases have occurred at the school, reinforcing the hypothesis of a causal relationship between environmental exposure to electromagnetic radiation and the emergence of the cluster.

Despite this, the official epidemiological studies commissioned by the Regional Government of Castile and León — particularly the report from the Carlos III Institute of Health, which was presented six years late despite repeated requests — analysed the cases by place of residence rather than by shared exposure at the school. This methodology was strongly criticised by families, associations and independent experts for diluting the clearly localised epidemiological pattern within a shared environment.

The case received wide media coverage at the time, although some content — such as the documentary *A contracorriente* ("Against the Current"), produced by *Documentos TV* (Spanish National Television, TVE), which included revealing testimonies and critical analyses of the situation — was never broadcast.

The Valladolid Association of People Affected by Telecommunications Antennas (AVAATE), which continues its work of public awareness and advocacy, considers this case to be one of the most serious examples in Spain of a possible link between electromagnetic emissions and public health effects, marked by an insufficient institutional response and a lack of transparency.

5.6 Enlightening Similarities

The German authors H. Baumer and W. Sönning, referred to earlier (see Chapter 3), describe the similarities between natural *sferics* and the technologically generated radiofrequency radiations used in mobile telephony. Both share a common feature: they consist of low-frequency (ELF) pulses that interact with living organisms and with their internal intercellular communication systems (Baumer & Sönning, 2002). For this reason, numerous experts have warned that it is highly questionable — even irresponsible — to saturate the environment with low-frequency pulsed electromagnetic radiation without first conducting rigorous research into its possible effects.

Scientific advances in the study of non-thermal effects reinforce concerns about the risks associated with the massive deployment of wireless technologies, both in civilian and military contexts. Furthermore, there has been a documented increase in the incidence of electromagnetic hypersensitivity syndromes linked to exposure to these new pulsed fields, indicating a growing impact across broader segments of the population. The recent rise in electromagnetic pollution has led to what can be described as a true epidemic of electrosensitive (EHS) individuals worldwide — people who struggle to live normally in urban areas — a problem that continues to grow as we become increasingly immersed in this sea of waves produced by widespread technological expansion (Hallberg & Oberfeld, 2006).

It is particularly striking — and clinically concerning — that the symptoms reported by individuals with electromagnetic hypersensitivity (EHS) show a symptomatological pattern remarkably similar to that of meteoropathic syndromes described in medical meteorology (see Chapter 2). The similarity between these two sets of symptoms suggests the existence of shared physiological mechanisms, possibly related to the sensitivity of the central or autonomic nervous system to imperceptible yet physically measurable environmental stimuli. This coincidence reinforces the hypothesis that certain individuals may be especially vulnerable to artificial electromagnetic fields, just as some are to specific meteorological conditions. Hence, it is increasingly evident that an interdisciplinary approach is needed — one that links environmental medicine, neurology, bioelectromagnetics and medical meteorology — to understand and address these emerging syndromes with scientific rigour.

Artificial electromagnetic radiations, which are always polarised and generally include pulses within the ELF (extremely low frequency) band, expose humans to higher intensities than natural *sferics* and may be significantly more bioactive, producing more unpleasant health symptoms in EHS individuals (Panagopoulos & Balmori, 2017).

Walach *et al.* (2001) suggested that it might be clinically relevant that some patients who experience headaches triggered by meteorological factors also exhibit sensitivity to electromagnetic radiation emitted by various electronic devices, such as mobile phones. This possible association between headache onset and weather changes — analysed in detail in Chapter 4 — has been supported by subsequent studies, which confirm that many people suffering from such headaches tend to identify atmospheric variations as a common trigger (Becker, 2011). In our own work (Panagopoulos & Balmori, 2017), we proposed a plausible biophysical explanation for this relationship, based on a shared biological sensitivity to these subtle electromagnetic stimuli.

Research findings also coincide in showing that technologically generated electromagnetic radiation, pulsed in the ELF range, modifies human electroencephalogram (EEG) alpha and beta waves (Kramarenko & Tan, 2003), just as natural *sferics* do, as discussed in earlier chapters.

For all these reasons, in our study (Panagopoulos & Balmori, 2017) we proposed that the perception of *sferics* — which manifests as a range of symptoms in sensitive individuals — may represent a specific expression of electrohypersensitivity (EHS). In turn, we suggested that EHS could be understood as a new form of meteoropathy induced by the contemporary technological environment, since in both cases the underlying triggering factor is the same: low-frequency electromagnetic pulses. This interpretation allows for the integration of phenomena that, although traditionally treated separately, share a common physiological and environmental basis. It could be said that, to varying degrees, we are all potentially electrohypersensitive. The difference lies in the duration and intensity of exposure: prolonged exposure to artificial electromagnetic fields may be sufficient for this latent condition to manifest..

According to a recent study funded by the French Agency for Food, Environmental and Occupational Health & Safety (ANSES), led by Laurène Sonzogni of the French National Institute of Health and Medical Research (INSERM), electromagnetic hypersensitivity (EHS) may be related to the biological management of single- and double-strand DNA breaks (Sonzogni *et al.*, 2025).

News reports increasingly frequent, about these emerging conditions — often associated with non-specific symptoms — tend to avoid linking them, in the media, to any potential causes that might negatively affect key sectors of economic growth, such as the technology industry (see Chapter 7).

Electrohypersensitivity (EHS) is a complex condition that has increasingly reached the courts, mainly through disability claims — particularly in cases involving women. These are relatively recent disorders whose diagnosis remains uncertain. A newly published study (Lousada & Ron, 2024) examines the various aspects of the legal treatment of MCS (Multiple Chemical Sensitivity) and EHS from a gender perspective. The study concludes that, due to their recent medical recognition, the legal handling of MCS and EHS remains unsatisfactory within current legislation, which, given that these conditions disproportionately affect women, constitutes a form of gender inequality.

Mobile phone radiation increases significantly in enclosed metallic spaces (cars, trains and buses) because reflections amplify the signal — the so-called "resonance" or "bell effect" — exposing nearby users, much like passive smokers. Out of respect for others, mobile phones should not be used in close proximity to other people, particularly the elderly, pregnant women and children. Unfortunately, such recommendations are not being communicated to the public; instead, mobile network operators continue to insist on the harmlessness of both antennas and handsets, often targeting their advertising campaigns at the most vulnerable and least protected groups — adolescents and children.

The insatiable greed and unstoppable advance of this techno-enthusiasm — seemingly without end (GSM, DCS, UMTS, WLAN, Wi-Fi, DECT, Bluetooth, Wi-MAX, 5G) — resemble a kind of slow-cooked collective electromagnetic ritual. The strategic importance of this sector to GDP and to media revenues (especially through advertising) does the rest, silencing the press and binding the hands of public authorities, leaving public health measures shamefully deferred to economic interests (see Chapter 7).

6

LIVING ORGANISMS AS BIOINDICATORS OF THE HUMAN HABITAT

Humans have often relied on living organisms to detect possible alterations in ecosystems and within their own living environments. From lichens—highly sensitive to pollution due to their ability to accumulate toxic substances in their tissues—to birds that inhabit gardens and buildings, a wide range of organisms has been used as indicators of the quality of the human habitat.

Historically, animals have been employed to detect environmental hazards, as in the case of canaries in coal mines, which served as an early warning of the presence of toxic gases. These species, owing to their smaller size, shorter lifespan and greater sensitivity to environmental changes, tend to provide clearer warning signs. Moreover, unlike humans, they do not experience psychosomatic effects—such as anxiety over mobile phone masts and their potential impacts. Similarly, trees, because of their immobility and continuous exposure, are regarded as excellent biological indicators.

For more than twenty years, the author has studied the effects of mobile phone radiation on animals and trees, publishing twenty-five scientific papers as a means of indirectly assessing its possible impact on humans. Some of these studies, together with research conducted by scientists around the world, will be discussed in the following sections.

6.1 The Effects of Technological Radiation on Animals and Plants

Since the widespread expansion of wireless telecommunications in the 1990s, the deployment of mobile phone networks has led to an exponential increase in environmental exposure to electromagnetic radiation, specifically in the radiofrequency (microwave) range, affecting all living organisms. Current public health protection standards only take into account the short-term thermal effects of exposure; however, the biological effects of electromagnetic radiation are dose-dependent, with chronic long-term effects and substantial experimental evidence of non-thermal biological effects that remain largely ignored today. Animals and plants are of particular interest in detecting potential effects, as they cannot be blamed for fearing or having phobias of new technologies.

Until now, researchers have paid little attention to the potential damage caused by radiation from mobile phone masts to wildlife, to the extent that this type of electromagnetic pollution is not even considered in environmental impact assessments, which, logically, should be conducted as a prerequisite before the installation of such emitting devices.

Despite its remarkable expansion over the past two decades, scientific activity focusing on the effects of mobile phone masts on wildlife has been considerably limited compared to research into other human infrastructure impacts, such as roads, power lines, or wind turbines. The few studies conducted have focused primarily on the impact of collisions with animals, particularly in the United States, where communication towers tend to be very large and conspicuous. However, the major problem associated with these masts—the effects of non-ionising electromagnetic radiation—has been scarcely investigated. This form of environmental pollution, which is ubiquitous, even affects natural spaces protected under strict conservation laws (Balmori, 2015).

Regarding exposure to electromagnetic fields, as previously noted, the application of the precautionary principle is becoming increasingly urgent in order to protect both wildlife and, of course, humans from non-thermal environmental effects. It is necessary to establish monitoring mechanisms, implement drastic reductions in emission levels, and promote technological advances that ensure environmental safety. Otherwise, this new, pervasive, and invisible pollutant could undermine current efforts aimed at conserving wildlife species (Balmori, 2014).

Fifteen years ago, I published an article in *Electromagnetic Biology and Medicine* titled "Mobile Phone Mast Effects on Common Frog (*Rana temporaria*) Tadpoles: The City Turned into a Laboratory" (Balmori, 2010). In this study, we exposed frog eggs and tadpoles to electromagnetic radiation from several mobile phone masts located 140 metres away. The experiment lasted for two months, from the egg stage to an advanced tadpole stage before metamorphosis. In the exposed group (n = 70), we observed poor coordination of movements, asynchronous growth (resulting in both large and small tadpoles), and a high mortality rate (90%). By contrast, the control group (n = 70), kept under the same conditions but inside a Faraday cage, exhibited normal movement coordination, synchronous development, and a mortality rate of only 4.2%.

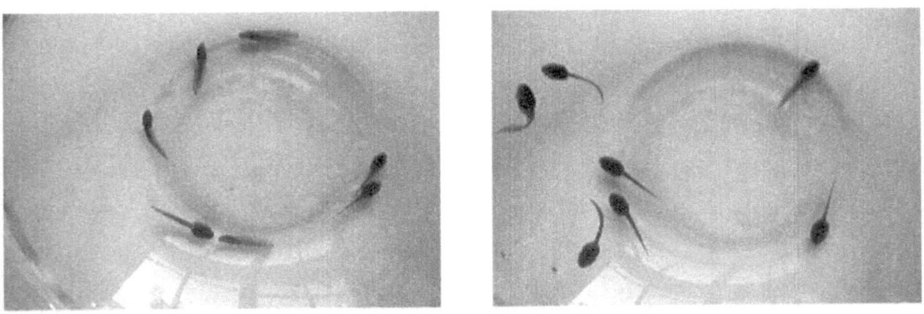

Figure 18: The experiment carried out with tadpoles. On the right, the group protected with a Faraday cage. On the left the exposed group. There is a clear difference in size and appearance of the tadpoles.

The results obtained indicate that radiation emitted by mobile phone masts, under real exposure conditions, affects the development of tadpoles and leads to increased mortality among the exposed specimens. These findings may have significant environmental implications, considering that the current environment is subjected to elevated levels of electromagnetic radiation from countless telecommunications masts. Despite being published fifteen years ago, this work has yet to be refuted by any scientist.

There is now sufficient scientific evidence to consider electromagnetic radiation as a risk to both the environment and human health. Numerous studies, conducted on animals and humans alike, have repeatedly demonstrated its adverse effects. Electromagnetic radiation should be recognised as an environmental pollutant capable of negatively impacting wildlife, which underscores the urgent need to open new lines of research and allocate dedicated resources for its study.

In a systematic review of the potential ecological effects of radiofrequency electromagnetic fields (RF-EMF) in the 10 MHz–3.6 GHz range, approximately two-thirds of the studies examined reported effects on living organisms, both at high and low levels of radiation (Cucurachi *et al.*, 2013). The "low" levels considered in these studies are comparable to those currently present in certain everyday environmental settings, both rural and urban. These results may have important implications for wildlife, particularly in urban and suburban areas, but also in rural zones and protected natural spaces where powerful radiofrequency emitters are often present.

Current evidence indicates that chronic exposure to electromagnetic radiation, at levels found in the environment, can particularly affect the immune, nervous, cardiovascular, and reproductive systems. Existing public health protection guidelines only account for short-term thermal effects and do not adequately safeguard wildlife. Animals exposed to emissions from nearby masts may experience health problems that disappear once they are moved away from the radiation source, with plausible cellular-level explanations for the observed effects (see Chapter 3). We will now outline some of the potential effects of human-generated electromagnetic radiation on wildlife.

6.1.1 Effects on Behaviour and Navigation (Orientation)

Different animal groups are sensitive to low-frequency electromagnetic fields, and many species possess receptor organs for natural electric fields that serve as important cues for orientation. Animals can use the direction of the Earth's magnetic field as a compass and its intensity as a navigational map, thanks to reactions occurring in specialised photopigments and to mechanisms involving tiny magnetite crystals within their bodies. They may rely on one or both of these systems, depending on the animal group in question. Insects and birds are particularly sensitive to electromagnetic fields and radiation.

The rapid development and increasing use of wireless telecommunication technologies have brought about a substantial change in exposure to radiofrequency electromagnetic fields. This increase in exposure has occurred mainly in outdoor areas due to emissions from mobile phone base stations. Current evidence suggests that exposure to levels commonly found in the environment—both in urban and rural areas with nearby base stations—can interfere with the receptor organs birds use to orient themselves in the Earth's magnetic field. However, the consequences of such interference for species conservation remain unknown (Balmori, 2015).

As with birds, radiofrequency fields also interfere with magnetoreception in insects. The geomagnetic field reception systems of the American cockroach are highly sensitive to radiofrequencies, which have a disruptive effect (Vácha *et al.*, 2009). For this reason, electromagnetic pollution should be regarded as a new problem affecting animal magnetoreception.

Insects use various senses for foraging, including the detection of visual cues such as colour and shape. However, they are also capable of perceiving electric fields generated by flowers—an additional sensory modality that enables rapid and dynamic communication between flowers and their pollinators. Some insects, such as bumblebees (*Bombus terrestris*), actively interact with these electric fields, and the ability to detect them represents a potentially significant form of sensory perception (Clarke *et al.*, 2013).

The ability of bees to perceive weak electric fields in nature represents a sensory modality that complements vision and smell, and it may have considerable adaptive value. Bees have also been shown to be sensitive to pulsed electromagnetic fields generated by devices such as mobile phones, which can induce changes in their behaviour (Favre, 2011; Odemer & Odemer, 2018).

These results could help explain the global decline in bee colonies recorded in recent years, a phenomenon known as *Colony Collapse Disorder* (CCD). Some authors argue that exposure to electromagnetic radiation provides a more convincing explanation than other proposed theories (Sainudeen Sahib, 2011; Cammaerts *et al.*, 2012). According to several studies, intense radiation generated by mobile phones and telecommunication antennas may interfere with the navigation system of bees, impairing their ability to return to the hive (Warnke, 2007; Sainudeen Sahib, 2011). Indeed, a correlation has been found between colony losses during winter in the north-eastern United States and the occurrence of geomagnetic storms (Ferrari, 2014). This new environmental pollutant has increased by several orders of magnitude and has become a global and ubiquitous problem that may play an important role in CCD (Balmori, 2009 and 2021; Bandara & Carpenter, 2018; Migdal *et al.*, 2025), either independently or acting synergistically with other factors

The migratory systems based on magnetoreception in some species, such as the monarch butterfly, may also be affected by anthropogenic radiofrequencies, which could represent a possible factor in the population decline experienced by this species. Radiofrequencies have also been shown to influence the behaviour of other invertebrates, such as ticks (Vargová *et al.*, 2017).

In an experimental electromagnetic field of approximately 1 V/m, results indicate that 900 MHz radiation (GSM, Global System for Mobile Communications) can seriously affect the nerve cells of exposed ants. In particular, deterioration was observed in visual and olfactory memory, together with a loss of the ability to use visual cues, which negatively influenced their orientation and navigation behaviour — functions essential for animals that rely on magnetic fields to move (Cammaerts *et al.*, 2012; Balmori, 2015). It is worth noting that this electric field intensity is even lower than that commonly encountered by these animals near mobile phone antennas. Therefore, insects could be used as bioindicators to detect and assess the biological effects of wireless technologies.

Radiofrequency fields in the megahertz range interfere with the fundamental processes of magnetoreception, thereby disabling the biological compass of birds and disrupting their orientation when such signals are present. For instance, it has been demonstrated that robins are unable to use their internal compass in the presence of radiofrequency pollution, as reported in Nature by German researchers from the University of Oldenburg (Engels *et al.*, 2014). Consequently, electromagnetic pollution directly affects the magnetic sensitivity of birds — a finding that should be seriously considered in the design and implementation of policies aimed at protecting the habitats of endangered species.

As we have seen, electromagnetic fields alter the activation of voltage-gated ion channels in cells (Panagopoulos *et al.*, 2000 and 2025; Pall, 2013). Moreover, when additional magnetic fields were applied to the cells of honeybees (*Apis mellifera*), changes were observed in the size of their magnetite granules, and these size alterations triggered increases in intracellular calcium levels (Hsu *et al.*, 2007). Therefore, we may hypothesise that some of the detrimental effects of radiofrequency fields on animal orientation could be related to interference with ion channels in cellular membranes. In habitats exposed to radiofrequency radiation (between 1–4 GHz), an aversive effect has also been found in bats (Nicholls & Racey, 2009).

Livestock exposed to 900 MHz radiofrequency emissions from nearby base stations may experience alterations in redox proteins and enzymatic activities. Furthermore, some animals appear to be sensitive to this radiation while others are not — a situation similar to that observed in humans (Hässig *et al.*, 2014). There is also scientific evidence indicating adverse effects of radiofrequency electromagnetic fields on the immune system, the pineal gland, circadian rhythms, oxidative stress, and teratogenicity (the occurrence of malformations).

Recently, my colleague Dimitris Panagopoulos proposed, in *Scientific Reports* (Nature Publishing Group), a new theory that unifies the causes of the biological effects of electromagnetic radiation on health and also on animal orientation through cellular ion channels (see Section 8.2) (Panagopoulos *et al.*, 2024). In that paper, he describes a biophysical mechanism for magnetoreception, orientation, and navigation in animals within the Earth's magnetic field, based on the forced oscillation mechanism of ions in voltage-gated ion channels of animal cell membranes. After reviewing previously suggested hypotheses, the authors argue that cellular ion channels are the most sensitive electromagnetic sensors in all animals. They demonstrate that animals with periodic variations in speed experience oscillating forces on their mobile ions within the ion channels, forcing them to oscillate and exerting forces on the voltage sensors of the channels that are comparable to, or greater than, the forces caused by membrane voltage changes that normally trigger activation. Consequently, the Earth's magnetic field, combined with variations in an animal's speed, can regulate cellular ion channels and alter cellular homeostasis to a degree that depends—given a specific speed and rate of change—on the intensity of the geomagnetic field (unique to each latitude) and on the angle between the animal's movement and the axis of the Earth's magnetic field, which determines its position and orientation.

6.1.2 Effects on Distribution and Habitat Loss

The distribution of a species refers to how its individuals are spread across a geographical area, while habitat loss involves the reduction, fragmentation, or alteration of the natural environment that a species requires to survive. Both aspects are closely interrelated, since changes in the environment—whether natural or induced by human activity—can profoundly modify where a species lives, and whether it can continue to exist in certain areas.

In the current context, a new and still poorly understood threat to wildlife is prolonged exposure to low-intensity electromagnetic radiation, such as that emitted by mobile phone base stations.

Studies conducted in Belgium and Spain have examined the possible effects of this radiation on populations of the house sparrow (*Passer domesticus*). The results reveal a consistent pattern: lower sparrow densities are found in areas where electromagnetic field intensity is higher (Balmori & Hallberg, 2007; Everaert & Bauwens, 2007). This suggests that these fields may influence the behaviour, physiology, or reproductive capacity of these birds, negatively affecting their persistence in certain urban environments.

This phenomenon has direct implications for the spatial distribution of sparrows. Where habitat conditions are altered by radiation—without visible changes such as tree felling or intensive urban development—birds may avoid the area or experience a gradual population decline. Over time, this can amount to a form of habitat loss, although not in the traditional sense. Instead of being displaced by physical destruction of their surroundings, species may be driven away by invisible yet significant changes in the ecological quality of their habitat.

In major cities such as London, a dramatic decline in sparrow populations has been recorded over the past two decades. Although this trend is likely to have multiple causes (including pollution, food scarcity, urbanisation, and climate change), the potential link between the proliferation of mobile phone antennas and the disappearance of these urban birds warrants deeper investigation. Electromagnetic radiation may be acting as a new type of environmental pollutant, exerting subtle but cumulative effects on the most sensitive species.

In summary, exposure to electromagnetic radiation may be contributing to a new, non-visible yet effective form of habitat loss. It represents an environmental alteration that reduces habitat suitability for certain species, affecting their geographical distribution and, in extreme cases, leading to local extinction. This type of impact highlights the importance of considering less obvious technological factors when studying the conservation of urban biodiversity. Section 6.2 will address in detail the specific case of sparrows and their worrying decline in many European cities.

6.1.3 Effects on Reproduction and Recruitment Rate

There is broad scientific consensus regarding the harmful effects of radiofrequency radiation on human and animal reproduction. Low-voltage power lines generate electromagnetic fields that negatively affect the reproductive success of birds such as the white stork (*Ciconia ciconia*), which often nest directly on electrical pylons (Vaitkuvienė & Dagys, 2014). Similar results have been found in nests exposed to radiofrequency radiation near mobile phone antennas — in other words, mobile phone masts interfere with the reproduction of storks.

To investigate these effects, a population of storks was monitored in Valladolid, Spain, in the vicinity of mobile phone antennas (Balmori, 2005). The total productivity in thirty nests located less than 200 metres from the antennas was 0.86 ± 0.16. In another thirty nests situated more than 300 metres away, productivity nearly doubled, with an average value of 1.6 ± 0.14. Twelve nests (40%) located within 200 metres of the antennas produced no chicks at all, whereas only one nest (3.3%) beyond 300 metres failed to produce offspring. The electric field intensity was significantly higher in nests within 200 metres of the antennas (2.36 ± 0.82 V/m) than in those more than 300 metres away (0.53 ± 0.82 V/m).

In locations less than 100 metres from one or more antennas, where the main radiation beam directly struck the nest, many chicks died from unknown causes (Balmori, 2005). Some storks that attempted to breed within 100 metres of the antennas, in the direction of the main emission beam, failed even to complete their nests. These results indicate that pulsed microwaves interfere with the reproduction of white storks, corroborating findings from laboratory-based research conducted by other authors..

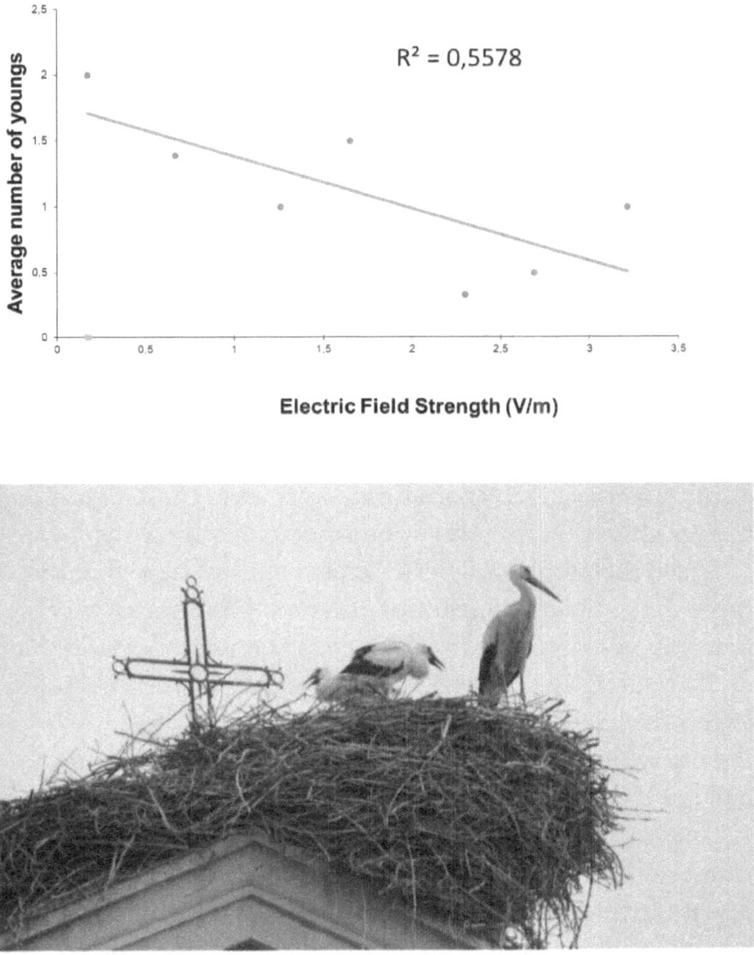

Figure 19: White storks (Ciconia ciconia) breeding at a distance from mobile phone antennas, with two chicks. Above, results from Balmori (2005) showing the inverse relationship between electric field strength and productivity in white storks.

Two years ago (in 2023), a team of researchers published an article entitled "Is there an effect of electromagnetic waves from base stations on the breeding success of *Ciconia ciconia* in Algeria?" (Sakraoui *et al.*, 2023). The fieldwork followed the methodological protocol previously established by the author in the study described above (Balmori, 2005). The aim of the Algerian study was to assess the effects of electromagnetic waves from mobile phone base stations on the reproduction of the white stork. To this end, the authors monitored the breeding phenology of storks according to the distance of their nests from mobile phone antennas over two consecutive breeding seasons, 2020 and 2021. The study was conducted in north-eastern Algeria, in the provinces of Annaba and El Tarf.

The nests were counted and divided into three distinct groups: the first comprised nests built directly on the repeater antennas; the second, nests located less than 200 metres away; and the third, nests situated more than 300 metres from the antennas. The authors evaluated nest occupancy, the average number of chicks per nest, and the proportion of nests without offspring. The results showed that nests located directly on the antennas had low reproductive success, as the majority (51.9%) produced no chicks. Those that did manage to rear chicks had smaller broods, not exceeding two nestlings. In contrast, the number of chicks tended to increase with distance from the base stations. Clutches of three or four chicks were generally found in nests more than 300 metres from mobile phone antennas.

In their analysis, the authors highlighted the concordance between their results and those reported by Balmori (2005), reinforcing the idea that a reduction in chick numbers constitutes a sensitive biological indicator of the effects of electromagnetic radiation.

The replication of scientific studies by independent research teams—as in this case, and in the study on sparrows that we shall discuss later—represents the most rigorous methodological standard for validating scientific results. Unfortunately, such important information is rarely, if ever, reported by mainstream media outlets.

Various studies conducted on different groups of animals have shown that exposure to microwave radiation similar to that emitted by mobile phone base stations causes abnormalities in mammalian sperm. Likewise, radiation emitted by mobile phones has been found to reduce ovarian development and cause DNA damage in certain insect species. Nonetheless, some supposedly scientific approaches continue to deny both the existence of evidence and the possibility that such radiation could affect human reproduction—an attitude that stands in stark contrast to the findings of most published studies on the subject (Adams *et al.*, 2014). In experimental laboratory studies, chicken eggs exposed to this type of radiation throughout the incubation period showed a significant increase in embryonic mortality (Batellier *et al.*, 2008).

6.1.4 Effects on Trees and Plants

A limited number of studies have examined the effects of radiofrequency radiation on plants, and indicate that these effects depend primarily on the plant family concerned, the stage of growth, the duration of exposure, the frequency, and the power density of the radiation, among other factors.

In tomato plants (*Lycopersicon esculentum*) exposed to an electric field strength of 5 V/m for a short period (ten minutes), changes were found in the abundance of three types of messenger RNA after exposure, as a direct consequence of the applied radiofrequency fields. The similarities in these responses suggest that such radiation is perceived by plants as a harmful stimulus, triggering cellular stress (Roux *et al.*, 2008).

Some years ago, we carried out long-term monitoring of trees (2006–2015) in the cities of Bamberg and Hallstadt (Germany), which we later published in *Science of the Total Environment* under the suggestive title: 'Radiofrequency radiation injures trees around mobile phone base stations' (Waldmann-Selsam *et al.*, 2016). To this end, we compiled a photographic record documenting unusual or unexplained damage to trees, accompanied by measurements of electromagnetic radiation levels. Many trees displayed damage patterns not attributable to harmful organisms—such as diseases (fungi, bacteria, viruses) and pests (insects, nematodes)—or to other environmental factors (water stress, heat, drought, frost, sunlight, soil compaction, or air and soil pollutants).

The main characteristics of the damage associated with radiation are as follows:

—Trees are affected predominantly on one side (showing unilateral differences and damage).
—Damage appears without external signs of infestation by insects, nematodes, fungi, bacteria, or viruses.
—Damage becomes evident one or two years after antenna installation, in trees that had previously grown well and were healthy.
—Over time, the damage progresses from the outer canopy towards the inner sections.
—Trees of different species located in the same area often exhibit similar types of damage.
—Damage occurs in both favourable locations (gardens, parks) and unfavourable ones, regardless of soil quality or other requirements.
—Trees situated in the same area but shielded by buildings or by other trees do not display damage.

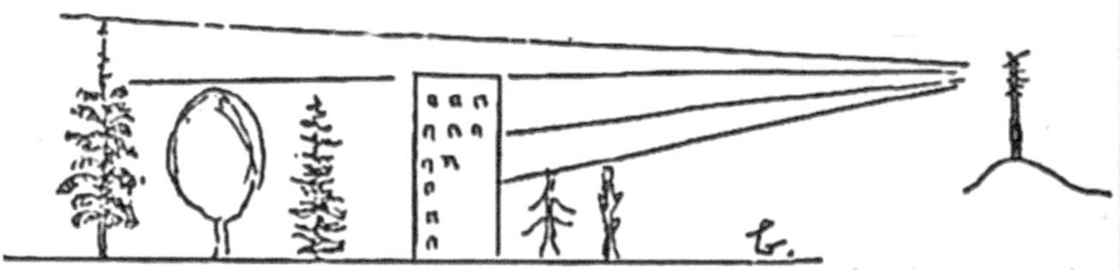

Figure 20. Drawing by Bernatzky (1986), clearly illustrating the damage caused by antennas to trees and the protection provided by obstacles positioned in front of the emission source.

—The number of leaves or needles decreases. The transparency of the crown increases from year to year.
—Leaves show premature discolouration, turning yellow, red, or brown.
—Premature leaf fall occurs.
—Over the years, the branches most affected by the radiation gradually dry out.
—The leader shoot of the tree often dies back (Figure 21).

—Trees exhibit irregular growth. They often stop growing upwards if doing so would expose them to higher levels of radiation (Figure 23).

The statistical analysis based on the field data demonstrated that electromagnetic radiation from mobile phone base stations is harmful to trees (Waldmann-Selsam *et al.*, 2016).

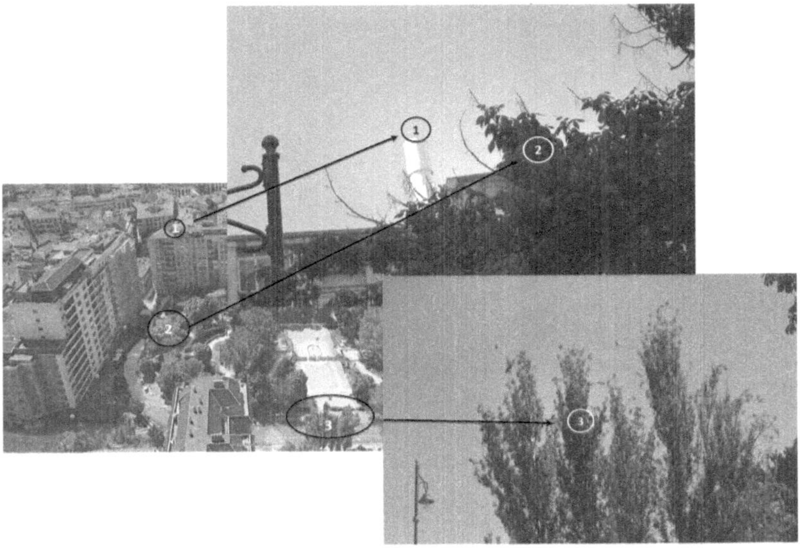

Figure 21. Typical examples of trees damaged in the vicinity of a mobile phone base station. 1: Camouflaged base station. 2: Acer negundo with all upper branches affected by radiation. 3: Populus alba specimens with dieback of the upper branches.

During medical examinations of individuals who had fallen ill while living near mobile phone base stations, damage was also observed in nearby trees (crown, leaves, trunk, branches, growth...), occurring simultaneously with the clinical symptoms. Evidence of radiation-related damage was found even in potted plants inside the homes of affected patients (Waldmann-Selsam *et al.*, 2016). Nearly ten years after the publication of this scientific paper, no one has been able to refute its results, yet unfortunately no measures have been taken to prevent the evident damage.

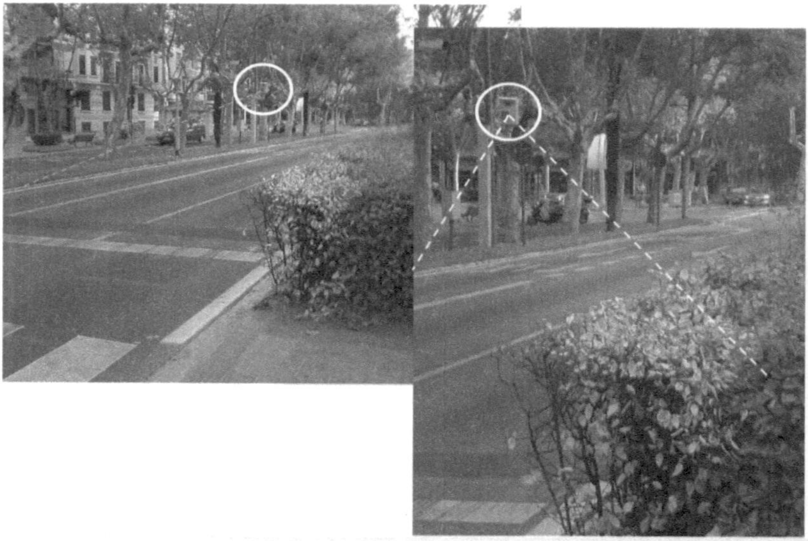

Figure 22. Clear effects on the Viburnum hedge in the central reservation, caused by radiation from a traffic radar.

On 18 February 2011, the first symposium on the effects of electromagnetic radiation on trees was held in the Netherlands, where noteworthy findings were presented demonstrating the disruptive effects of such radiation on them. These types of damage had been reported by the author of this book and published six years earlier in the journal *Ecosistemas* (Balmori, 2004).

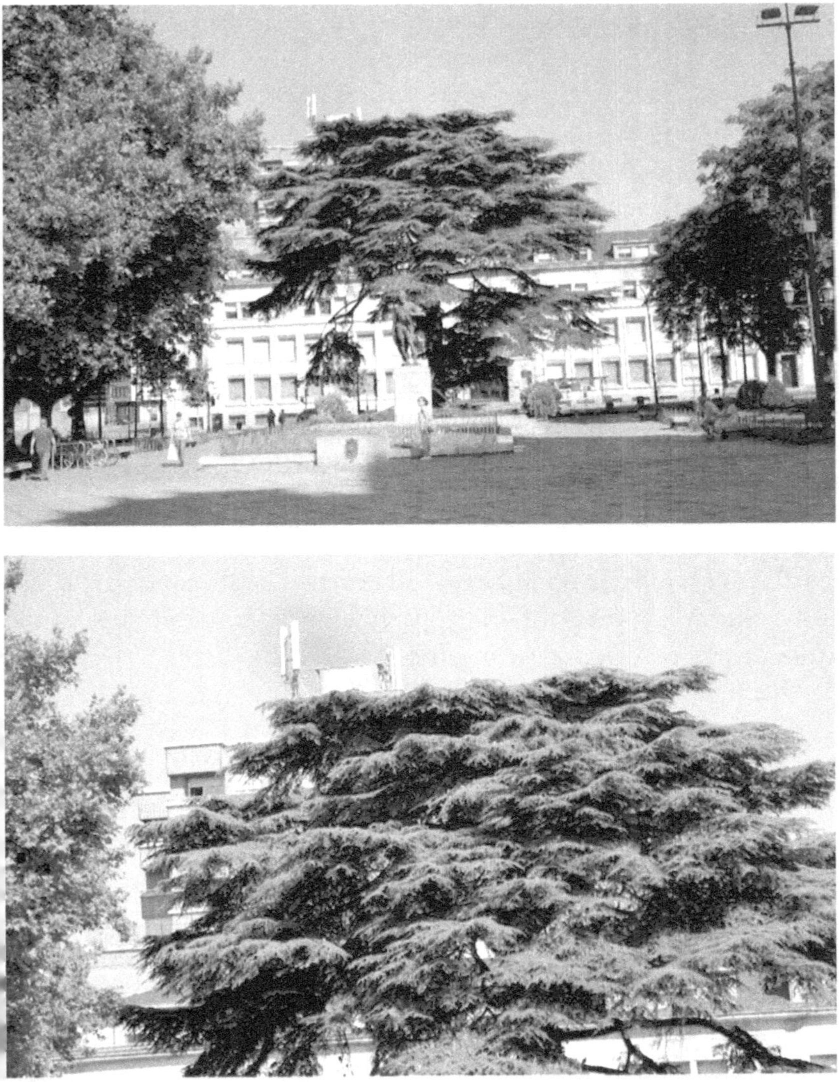

Figure 23. Lebanon cedar that ceased its apical growth twenty years ago.

6.2 Why Are Sparrows Disappearing from Cities?

The House Sparrow (*Passer domesticus*) is a species familiar to everyone, inhabiting urban and suburban environments, and it has spread from its original Eurasian range to numerous cities around the world. Over recent decades, a decline in House Sparrow populations has been observed in several European cities. In the United Kingdom, a 71% decrease was recorded in London between 1994 and 2002, and urban sparrow populations in the southeast of England are disappearing at a faster rate than rural ones. For this reason, the House Sparrow has been included on the UK Red List of Endangered Species. The decline of House Sparrow populations appears to be a widespread phenomenon across much of their European range (Mohring *et al.*, 2020). In Brussels, Ghent and Antwerp, many sparrow populations have vanished, and similar decreases have been reported in Dublin. In Spain, in a study carried out between 1998 and 2008, the abundance of House Sparrows fell by around 70% in the urban parks of Valencia (Murgui & Macías, 2010).

The most comprehensive and recent study was conducted in Paris, analysing fine-scale habitat characteristics and population trends of House Sparrows over fifteen years (2003–2017), at 200 different sites across the city (Mohring *et al.*, 2020). The results show a drastic 89% decline in sparrows during the study period, which was most pronounced in locations that had held the largest numbers of sparrows at the start of the study.

However, the decline in sparrow numbers is not confined to Europe. In India, their numbers have dropped sharply in several parts of the country (Singh *et al.*, 2013; Shende & Patil, 2015). These worldwide reductions are a cause for concern, as House Sparrows generally inhabit cities and suburban areas and serve as important bioindicators of the health of urban ecosystems, acting as an urban sentinel species for humans.

Despite numerous studies attempting to explain this decline, there is still no robust theory that resolves the underlying causes of the phenomenon, although several hypotheses have been proposed to date. In 2021, I published an article in the journal *Birds*, arguing that there is strong evidence that the global increase in electromagnetic radiation—particularly in cities—may be playing a role, in combination with other previously discussed factors, in the species' decline.

6.2.1 Hypotheses Proposed to Explain the Decline of the House Sparrow

The most important explanatory hypotheses put forward so far are the following:

—Lack of food in urban areas affecting both nestlings and adults; in particular, a shortage of insects, which adults rely on to feed their young.
—Cleaner streets resulting in fewer foraging opportunities.
—Competition for food with other urban species.
—Increased predation by domestic cats.
—Increased pressure from predators due to a possible recovery of urban populations of the Eurasian Sparrowhawk (*Accipiter nisus*).
—Loss of nesting sites because newly built houses often lack suitable cavities for the species.
—Greater use of pesticides in parks and gardens.
—Pollution.
—Transmission of diseases.

For many authors, this situation may be attributed to several interacting and cumulative effects.

However, in the study carried out in Paris mentioned earlier (Mohring *et al.*, 2020), House Sparrows were not genuinely lacking nesting sites. They also declined everywhere, and trends in their abundance were independent of habitat characteristics; even areas with extensive green spaces failed to provide sufficient quality to maintain large populations. Furthermore, in Paris, Sparrowhawks (*Accipiter nisus*) bred for the first time in 2008, when House Sparrows were already clearly in decline, so this factor is not considered explanatory either.

On the other hand, it is well known that pollution (air quality) can cause negative physiological effects, such as increased oxidative stress, and adversely affect sparrow reproduction. The authors of the Paris study examined the evolution of eighteen atmospheric pollutants in the city during the study period (2003–2017) and related them to House Sparrow abundance. They found that the highest figures were recorded at the beginning of the period, when air pollution was at its peak, and that no deterioration in air quality occurred during the fifteen years analysed. For this reason, they concluded that atmospheric pollution was not responsible for the observed decline, nor were meteorological fluctuations.

The authors explain that their study did not assess the potential influence of other specific urban disturbances previously proposed as possible causes, such as increasing noise, light, and/or electromagnetic pollution. Nor did they examine the influence of the rising abundance of domestic cats (the other major sparrow predator), increasing interspecific competition with other urban exploiters, or the presence of diseases and parasites (Mohring *et al.*, 2020). Indeed, another, more recent study showed that avian malaria (*Plasmodium relictum*) has a higher prevalence in London sparrows and may be contributing to the species' declining trend (Dadam *et al.*, 2019).

6.2.2 Electromagnetic Radiation as a Probable Factor

In Flanders, Belgium, the potential effect of prolonged exposure to low-intensity electromagnetic radiation emitted by mobile phone base stations (GSM) on the number of House Sparrows during the breeding season was investigated (Everaert & Bauwens, 2007). The study was carried out by sampling 150 points across six different areas to examine small-scale geographical variation in the number of male sparrows, while simultaneously measuring the intensity of electromagnetic radiation emitted by mobile phone masts. Spatial variation in sparrow numbers was negatively correlated with the electric field strength of mobile phone signals (900 and 1800 MHz frequency bands). This negative correlation was very similar in each of the six study areas, despite substantial differences between them both in bird numbers and radiation levels. Thus, the study demonstrated that sparrow numbers correlate with levels of electromagnetic pollution, and it supports the idea that long-term exposure to high levels of radiation adversely affects the abundance or behaviour of wild House Sparrows (Everaert & Bauwens, 2007).

In another similar study, conducted by the author of this book (the Belgian researchers from the previous study contacted him to learn about the methodology he was using), thirty sampling points were established in the city of Valladolid. These points were visited monthly over more than three years (n = 40 censuses in total), recording sparrow numbers and measuring average electric field strength (radiofrequencies and microwaves in the range 1 MHz to 3 GHz). The results showed that bird density was significantly lower in areas with high levels of electromagnetic pollution, and a general decline in bird density over time was also detected (Balmori & Hallberg, 2007).

Two studies carried out in India likewise show that sparrows are disappearing from areas with mobile phone masts, where electromagnetic pollution is highest (Singh *et al.*, 2013; Shende & Patil, 2015). The first study involved monthly monitoring of urban and rural areas and revealed that House Sparrow populations were rapidly disappearing in areas contaminated with electromagnetic radiation, particularly in urban zones where phone masts are more common (Shende & Patil, 2015). The second study lasted two years and selected rural sites with abundant nesting opportunities, food, water and roosting sites, and with a low risk of predation. In such areas, the population should have increased; however, the author observed a decline. Notably, the most marked reduction in nests occurred at sites with the greatest number of operational mobile phone masts, leading the author to propose electromagnetic radiation as the probable cause (Singh *et al.*, 2013).

A shortage of invertebrate prey during the breeding season, which is used to feed nestlings, has also been suggested as a possible explanation for the population decline of House Sparrows in urban centres (Summers-Smith, 2003), as the availability of key insect prey such as *Aphidoidea*, *Curculionidae*, *Orthoptera* and *Lepidoptera* is essential for nestling growth and development. Numerous studies have shown that electromagnetic pollution may affect insect abundance (see section 6.3), reducing the availability of the insects with which House Sparrows feed their young (Balmori, 2021).

The studies reviewed and analysed indicate that electromagnetic radiation is not only a plausible factor but a probable one, for multiple reasons, including the fact that it is the only factor involved in all other hypotheses proposed to date. Electromagnetic radiation is a form of pollution that affects chick productivity, negatively influences fertility, reduces insect populations (Lázaro *et al.*, 2016), causes habitat loss and impairs the immune system (Galeev, 2000). It is well known that a stressed immune system can increase birds' susceptibility to infectious diseases, bacteria, viruses and parasites.

6.2.3 Effects of Electromagnetic Radiation on Other Bird Species

There are several noteworthy studies that investigate the response of urban birds in relation to their distance from mobile phone masts, as electric field strength is determined by this distance (Balmori, 2009).

Several studies conducted in India examined the presence of different bird species near mobile phone masts. Most birds were found in areas with lower radiation levels, and no bird nests were detected close to the masts (Bhattacharya & Roy, 2014). In another study, the presence of birds in exposed and non-exposed areas was 28.08% and 71.91%, respectively (Bose *et al.*, 2020). A third study found that the number of birds recorded within a 200 m radius of a mobile phone base station was lower than that recorded outside this radius (Bhat & Singh, 2019).

The studies mentioned above indicate that birds disappear from areas most contaminated by electromagnetic radiation. Furthermore, there are studies addressing the impact of radiation on other animals, as well as laboratory investigations demonstrating its effects at electric field intensities comparable to those present in urban environments.

Considered together, the results of all these studies support the hypothesis that electromagnetic pollution may be responsible—either alone or in combination with other factors—for the reduction in sparrow numbers in cities in recent years. Moreover, the disappearance of sparrows and the introduction of mobile phone masts are temporally correlated: the decline of sparrows coincides chronologically with the deployment of mobile phone networks, particularly over the last few decades. Additionally, the mechanisms underlying the non-thermal effects of electromagnetic radiation that could affect sparrows and contribute to their decline are well understood.

Therefore, electromagnetic radiation should be taken seriously as a factor in the decline of House Sparrows, probably acting in synergy with the other factors proposed above. Indeed, the study conducted in Paris suggests that specific environmental changes have taken place in the city during the last fifteen years and that current conditions are unsuitable for maintaining dense local populations of House Sparrows (Mohring, 2020).

6.3 The Marked Decline of Insects

6.3.1 The Importance of Insects and Their Ecosystem Services

Numerous studies demonstrate the fundamental importance of insects as keystone species within ecosystems. Some of the most significant ecosystem services they provide include climate regulation, crop pollination, agricultural pest control, and seed dispersal. In addition, decomposer insects (also known as detritivores or saprophages) recycle nutrients within ecosystems by feeding on dead organic matter (such as plant and animal remains, faeces, etc.), releasing the nutrients they contain and making them available once again to plants and other organisms, thus completing the nutrient cycle.

For these reasons, insects form the structural and functional foundation of many of the world's ecosystems, and they also constitute the primary food base for numerous birds, reptiles, amphibians and bats.

6.3.2 The Current Decline of Insects and Its Causes

A study carried out by monitoring insects colliding with car windscreens in rural areas of Denmark, using data collected between 1997 and 2017, concluded that insect numbers had declined by 80% over those twenty years. The authors attributed this decrease primarily to modern agricultural practices and the use of pesticides (Møller, 2019).

After reviewing seventy-three historical reports on insect declines worldwide, another study revealed that insect biodiversity is globally threatened, and current rates of decline could lead to the extinction of 40% of species. According to the results of this review, the groups most affected are *Lepidoptera* (butterflies), *Hymenoptera* (bees and ants), and *Coleoptera* (beetles) in terrestrial ecosystems, and *Odonata* (dragonflies), *Plecoptera*, *Trichoptera* (caddisflies) and *Ephemeroptera* (mayflies) in aquatic systems. The authors conclude that the main plausible causes, in order of importance, are the following: habitat loss, especially due to intensive agricultural change and urbanisation; pollution, mainly from pesticides and synthetic fertilisers; introduced invasive species; and climate change (Sánchez-Bayo & Wyckhuys, 2019).

Furthermore, several studies have found evidence of declines across a large proportion of pollinator species. The reduction of pollinators may have significant ecological and economic impacts, potentially affecting the maintenance of wild plant diversity, agricultural production and human well-being (Lázaro *et al.*, 2016). The loss of insect diversity and abundance triggers cascading effects on food webs and ecosystem services (Møller, 2019).

6.3.3 Electromagnetic Radiation May Be Contributing to the Decline

Insects are particularly sensitive to electromagnetic radiation. An increasing number of reports indicate that flies and spiders, among other invertebrates, are disappearing from areas receiving the highest levels of radiation from mobile phone masts. These observations are consistent with numerous studies demonstrating negative effects of electromagnetic radiation on reproductive success, development and orientation (Balmori, 2021; Lázaro *et al.*, 2016).

Evidence of the non-thermal effects of electromagnetic radiation has been known for fifty years. One study showed that the reproductive capacity of fruit flies decreased by 50–60% after exposure to the radiofrequency signal of a mobile phone during the first two to five days of adult life (Panagopoulos *et al.*, 2004). Belgian researchers experimentally demonstrated the effect of 900 MHz electromagnetic waves on the olfactory and visual learning of ants, as their speed and movements were immediately altered by the presence of these waves (Cammaerts *et al.*, 2012).

In several studies conducted in natural habitats containing actual mobile phone masts, electromagnetic radiation (EMR) emitted by telecommunications antennas affected the abundance and composition of wild pollinator communities (Lázaro *et al.*, 2016). In another study investigating the effects of mobile phone masts on the distribution, diversity and abundance of several groups of insects, carried out in Nigeria, the intensity of electromagnetic radiation and the number of pollinating insects were monitored daily over twenty-two weeks. Radiation intensity was found to have negative effects on the distribution, diversity and abundance of insects in these areas (Adelaja *et al.*, 2021). Another study warned that the shorter wavelengths used by the new generations of mobile telecommunications (5G) are comparable to the body size of insects and are therefore expected to increase radiation absorption in this group (Thielens *et al.*, 2018).

Another important study, recently published in the prestigious journal *Science Advances*, assessed the effect of electromagnetic fields on the pollination efficiency of bees through field and laboratory experiments. It was observed that exposure induces physiological stress in bees, altering the expression of behaviour-related genes. In addition, California poppy plants located near the radiation source received fewer bee visits and produced fewer seeds. Finally, it was found that electromagnetic fields negatively affect plant species richness and abundance. The study concludes that electromagnetic fields have detrimental effects on bee pollination and, consequently, on plant communities (Molina-Montenegro *et al.*, 2023).

As shown by most of the research carried out to date, EMR can pose a problem for insects and for their orientation, and both laboratory and field analyses with different invertebrate species have demonstrated this. Electromagnetic radiation should therefore be taken seriously as an additional factor contributing to the dramatic decline of insects, acting in synergy with agricultural intensification, pesticides, invasive species and climate change. The extent to which anthropogenic electromagnetic radiation represents a significant threat to pollinating insects remains both unresolved and plausible. For these reasons, and considering the benefits insects provide to nature and to humanity, the precautionary principle should be applied before any new deployment.

6.3.4 Our Systematic Review

In 2024, together with Central European researchers, we published a systematic review of all studies conducted on the effects of electromagnetic radiation on insects (Thill *et al.*, 2024). The vast majority reported effects—generally harmful—and it is unlikely that these findings are the result of chance. The existence of consistent results across numerous studies carried out by different research groups, using different protocols, constitutes irrefutable evidence of the adverse effects of electromagnetic fields on insects.

Thirty-six of the fifty-five studies on high-frequency electromagnetic fields included in the review used field intensities below 6 V/m (~100 mW/m^2), and thirty-one of these thirty-six (86%) nevertheless found statistically significant adverse effects, beginning at approximately 2 V/m and reaching a maximum at around 6 V/m. These levels are far below the regulatory thresholds established by the International Commission on Non-Ionizing Radiation Protection (ICNIRP) (41 V/m or 61 V/m above 2 GHz), and even below the particularly strict limits found in only a few countries (the installation limit is measured in places where people may remain for long periods of time, such as homes, schools, workplaces and children's play areas). These findings of biological effects on insects, from around 2 V/m, imply that current standards should be revised and made more stringent, so as to incorporate concerns regarding the protection of nature and wildlife.

6.4 The Enigma of Mass Strandings of Live Cetaceans

One of the most intriguing mysteries for the scientific community and for marine mammal specialists is that of mass strandings: the unexpected appearance of dozens or even hundreds of still-living individuals, agonising on the shore. These events often involve healthy animals which, for reasons unknown, return repeatedly towards the coast despite repeated attempts by rescue teams to guide them back out to sea.

The species that suffer most from these mass events are pilot whales, although the problem also affects dolphins, porpoises, sperm whales and the majority of odontocetes (toothed whales). Their high degree of sociability appears to play an important role in these episodes, since in the more solitary group of mysticetes (which includes the large baleen whales), strandings are seldom mass events and usually involve only a small number of individuals.

There are strandings with clearly identified causes, directly linked to human activities, such as those associated with fishing operations (for instance, accidental bycatch and entanglement in fishing nets). Larger species tend to fall victim to vessel collisions, whereas smaller species may become entangled in fishing gear. Other causes include hunting; naval manoeuvres; sonar operations that cause auditory disturbance; acoustic trauma from dynamite use; seismic surveys carried out primarily by the oil and gas industry; and the toxicity of certain marine pollutants.

However, strandings also occur for entirely natural reasons, without human involvement. In such cases, possible causes include disorientation, injury or illness—*Morbillivirus* infections are relatively common in striped dolphins (*Stenella coeruleoalba*) and pilot whales (*Globicephala melas*). Other episodes have been linked to parasitism, harmful algal blooms and predator attacks. Additional proposed causes include coastal configuration, oceanographic events, topographical factors, turbulent weather, navigational errors, wind anomalies, climate change, or alterations in prey distribution and availability.

Nevertheless, the question that has long remained unresolved—and continues to generate uncertainty among scientists and environmentalists—is what precisely lies behind the mass strandings of live cetaceans, particularly in cases where no obvious or conclusive cause has been identified to explain such unusual behaviour.

6.4.1 Our Proposal

At the end of December 2023, we published a scientific article reviewing the different causes of mass strandings of live cetaceans and proposing a new hypothesis for this serious conservation problem affecting marine mammals (Balmori-de la Puente & Balmori, 2024). We suggested that anthropogenic radiofrequency radiation (RFR), emitted by radar systems, could interfere with cetacean orientation and communication—especially in odontocetes, which are far more social—thereby playing some role in mass strandings of live cetaceans, for which no plausible explanations have yet been found.

As we have seen throughout this book, anthropogenic electromagnetic fields represent a little-known yet potentially important emission source, which is increasing in both terrestrial and marine environments, altering or masking environmental signals vital for species sensitive to them (Hutchison *et al.*, 2020). Some authors have warned that anthropogenic electromagnetic fields constitute the fastest-growing form of environmental pollution (Levitt & Lai, 2010; Balmori, 2014) and may pose a threat to wildlife orientation (Balmori, 2015). Important recent reviews have also been published on the effects of technologically generated electromagnetic fields on animals, including mammals (Levitt *et al.*, 2022).

To attempt to test our hypothesis, we carried out an extensive literature review of the scientific articles dealing with mass strandings of live cetaceans. At the same time, we conducted searches in publicly accessible databases of military and meteorological radar systems worldwide, using the following sources:

—https://www.radars.org.uk/ (military radars)
—https://wrd.mgm.gov.tr/Home/Wrd (meteorological radars)

We considered the timeline of the installation of military and meteorological radar systems across the world, together with cetacean strandings over the years, to identify potential links with mass strandings of unknown cause. The aim was to detect temporal or spatial patterns in clusters of strandings along coastlines, or recurrent spatial concentrations in specific locations. Finally, to determine whether anthropogenic RFR from military and meteorological radars could have played a role in any of these strandings, we performed a linear regression analysis between the cumulative number of radar installations and strandings with or without known causes in the United Kingdom, where records are the most systematic. This analysis combined the military radar dataset for the period 1913–2015 with the strandings recorded during the same period (Coombs *et al.*, 2019).

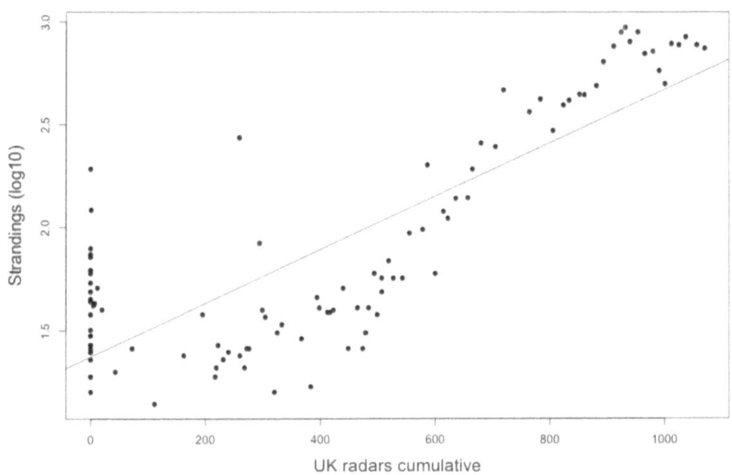

***Figure 24:** Linear regression between the cumulative number of military radar installations in the United Kingdom over one hundred years (from 1913 to 2015) and the number of cetacean strandings.*

The literature review revealed numerous studies showing an increase in the number of cetacean strandings in recent decades, although it is still unclear whether this rise is influenced by improved detection capabilities due to greater human presence and coastal monitoring in recent times. In North America and the United Kingdom, there has been a sharp increase in the number of stranding reports since 1970, and especially since 1990, likely due to intensified fishing activities but also to public efforts to report strandings.

The upward trend in stranding numbers is widespread. A continuous increase in strandings has been observed throughout the 20th century along the coasts of the United Kingdom and Ireland, particularly from the 1970s and 1980s, and between 2002 and 2014. In the Philippines, there is also a general upward trend in strandings since 2004, with no known cause. Along the Galician coast (Spain), there is a clear increase in the analysis of live or recently deceased specimens, but the greater human presence monitoring the coasts does not fully explain this trend (López *et al.*, 2002). In Western Australia, recorded mortality of stranded humpback whales (*Megaptera novaeangliae*) is also rising, and this increase is independent of the number of observers (Coughran *et al.*, 2013). Reports of cetacean strandings in Chile have risen steadily, especially over the past twenty years, with the authors of the study and monitoring urging immediate action to understand the unknown causes of this phenomenon (Alvarado-Rybak *et al.*, 2020).

At the same time, since the Second World War, numerous military air and naval radars have been installed along coasts worldwide, and more recently, many meteorological radars have been added (Figure 25).

In our study, we identified a total of thirty-one articles in the scientific literature reporting on clusters of strandings with no known cause over time and space. These studies were carefully evaluated to identify radars in their vicinity (~50 km), using public databases and visual inspections of these areas with Google Earth. Radars were found nearby in 65% (20 out of 31) of these stranding cases.

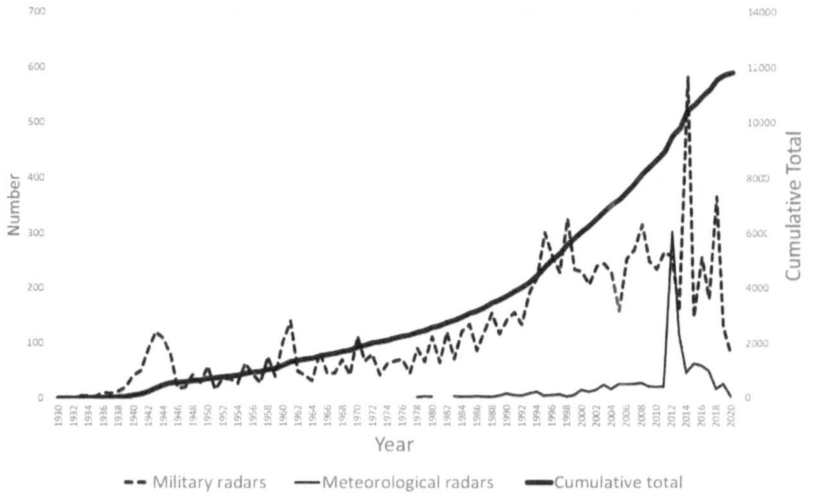

Figure 25: Global numerical evolution of the number of radars.

Regarding the spatial concentration of strandings, we found seven articles showing clear patterns of increased stranding concentrations along the coast following the installation of a radar. Therefore, we observed an accumulation of strandings in different areas of the world after radar installation (black points). Additionally, further temporal evidence was found, as in several of the areas studied there was a clear increase in strandings from the date of radar installation.

Although it might be argued that radar waves do not affect cetaceans because they live underwater, it is well known that radio frequencies can penetrate water to a certain depth. For example, other electromagnetic radiations with shorter wavelengths, such as visible light, penetrate tens of metres into the water in the photic zone. Moreover, many cetacean species, such as pilot whales or dolphins, spend a considerable amount of time at the surface, with part of their bodies out of the water due to their mode of movement and the need to breathe.

Therefore, the existence of a relationship between radar installation and the occurrence of mass strandings of live specimens is plausible.

6.4.2 Magnetoreception in Cetaceans and Its Possible Implications

There is growing evidence that the magnetic sense plays an important role in cetacean orientation and migration, and that live strandings are associated with anomalies in the Earth's magnetic field. A plausible explanation for such live strandings is therefore the disorientation of migrating cetaceans, triggered by solar storms that disrupt the geomagnetic field as variable energy flows reach the Earth from the Sun. Sunspots are strongly correlated with solar storms (which we shall examine in Chapter 9), and it has been shown that radio frequencies reaching the Earth from these storms are closely linked to the strandings of grey whales (*Eschrichtius robustus*) (Granger *et al.*, 2020).

6.4.3 Anthropogenic Radio Frequencies May Have the Same Effects as Those Originating from the Sun

Research carried out on migratory birds has shown that radio frequencies directly interfere with the primary processes of magnetoreception and disable the birds' magnetic compass while they are present. Other researchers have confirmed that migratory birds are unable to use their magnetic compasses in the presence of urban electromagnetic noise, and that anthropogenic radio-frequency electromagnetic fields disrupt the functioning of their sensory systems (Engels *et al.*, 2014). Radio-frequency electromagnetic noise also disorientates mice and arthropods (Phillips *et al.*, 2022; Vácha *et al.*, 2009).

Therefore, given current knowledge about the interference that RFR causes in the magnetoreception process, it is plausible that human-installed radars (which operate in the order of a few GHz) could disorientate cetaceans and in some way contribute to mass strandings of live individuals.

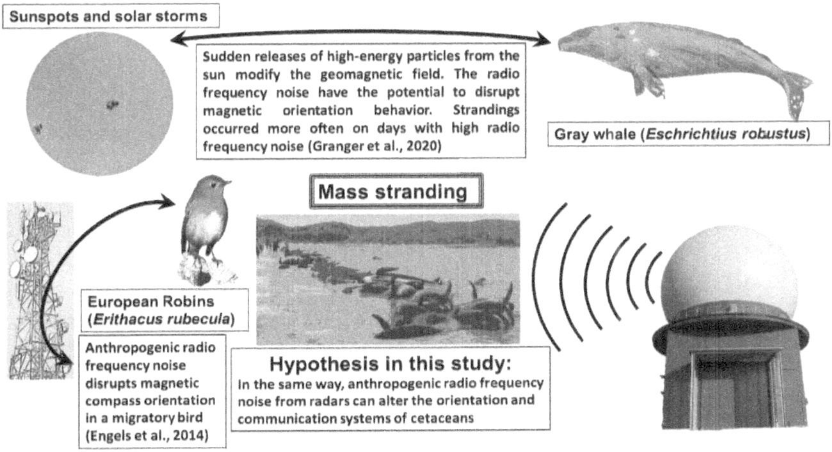

Figure 26: Hypothesis proposed in our work, taking into account the studies by Granger et al. (2020) and Engels et al. (2014).

6.4.4 Mechanisms of Action

Radar repeatedly emits short-duration pulses, while the carrier wave is a radio-frequency signal. There are several ways in which radio-frequency pulses from radar systems could lead to strandings.

—The thermoelastic expansion mechanism. Human auditory perception of pulsed radio frequencies has been reported since the 1940s, and may result from the thermoelastic expansion mechanism (Foster & Finch, 1974). Cetaceans may be highly sensitive to the thermoelastic effects of radar pulses—possibly even more so than humans—as they can perceive pulses that are much closer together in time, even when the interval between pulses is only a few milliseconds.

—Delphinid vocalisations. Delphinid vocalisations fall into two functional categories: echolocation clicks, used for navigation and orientation in the ocean, and pulsed sounds and frequency-modulated whistles, used for communication (social signals). Cetaceans can use high-frequency pulses (50–200 kHz) to detect prey, whereas lower-frequency pulses (down to 20

Hz) are preferred for communication and navigation. Radar pulses could therefore interfere with both the echolocation and communication systems of these animals.

—Interference with echolocation systems. Odontocetes use echolocation for both prey detection and navigation. For instance, dolphins possess a highly developed auditory system—arguably the most advanced among animals. They can hear across a wide range of frequencies and are remarkably capable of perceiving extremely short signals lasting only tens of microseconds. The specific characteristics of the cochlea and auditory nervous system suggest a particular need for fine detail and rapid processing of acoustic information in the aquatic environment, where sound travels faster than in air.

—Interference with the pulsed communication systems of odontocetes. All odontocetes produce characteristic pulsed sounds in rapid bursts, with a high repetition rate (>300 pulses per second) or short interpulse intervals (<3 ms). Radar may mimic these communication pulses and cause confusion in more social species such as odontocetes. As we have seen, odontocetes are the group most frequently involved in mass strandings of live animals. Such interference with their own communication systems could help explain the persistent tendency of stranded groups to return repeatedly to the shore—something commonly observed when rescue teams attempt to guide animals back into deeper waters.

—Other known mechanisms of low-frequency pulsed radio-frequency action. Some disruptive effects may be associated with the opening of voltage-gated calcium channels in cells, as well as interference with brain waves, as discussed in previous chapters. Notably, studies on bats (which also use echolocation to forage) have shown that electromagnetic radiation associated with radar installations can elicit behavioural responses that deter these animals from approaching them (Nicholls & Racey, 2007).

It would be presumptuous and methodologically unsound to attribute mass cetacean strandings solely to the influence of electromagnetic radiation. Nevertheless, dismissing its potential relevance in advance—within the broad range of factors that may contribute to this complex phenomenon—would be equally unscientific and reductionist, running counter to the spirit of rigorous and open-minded inquiry.

7
WHEN SCIENCE COLLIDES WITH ECONOMICS

7.1 Conflicts of Interest

As we have seen in the preceding chapters, living beings (and certainly human beings) are extremely sensitive to artificial electromagnetic radiation that affects our cells and organs in one way or another, just as natural *sferics* originating in the atmosphere and in earthquakes, or solar radiation, do (Chapters 8 and 9).

There are powerful official reasons not to support further research into the effects of electromagnetic radiation on living organisms. In a society overly focused on the economic growth of large corporations, studies, research, or opinions that contradict the official narrative are ignored, dismissed, or silenced. Research that favours market forces (that which promises greater commercial opportunity and profitability) tends to be given greater prominence and publicity—leading to wider social impact—while findings that run counter to those interests may even be actively suppressed, even when adverse effects on health may exist (Hyland, 2001).

And it is not merely that, in the rush to make this new and valuable technology widely available, the necessary research into its safety has been set aside or abandoned; it is rather that—far more reprehensibly—the signs that already pointed to its potential risks have been, and continue to be, carefully and deliberately ignored, both by the industry itself and by national and international regulatory bodies (Hyland, 2001).

This is precisely what is happening with the numerous studies warning of an increase in brain tumours among mobile-phone users, specifically in the regions of the brain where radiation penetrates most deeply. The gravest charge that can be levelled against a mobile phone is that it tears out pages from the book in which the secret of life is written—the codes that make life possible. Mutations in DNA are the first step in the development of tumours and neurodegenerative diseases. Yet, for those of us who have followed closely the "hijacking of science" and the scandal that has been taking shape around this field of research for far too many years, these results offer little that is genuinely new. Although industry and some authorities have systematically ignored them, it can be stated that the radiation emitted by mobile phones at current power-density levels has genotoxic effects.

Traditionally, it had been considered impossible for non-ionising radiation at low power densities to produce such effects. Yet these findings are not new: Henry Lai's team at the Bioelectromagnetics Research Laboratory (Department of Bioengineering, University of Washington) published exactly this thirty years ago, when mobile-phone networks were only beginning to be rolled out (Lai and Singh, 1995). This discovery does not necessarily imply harm to the health of exposed humans or animals, since the body's cells possess efficient DNA-repair systems. Unfortunately, however, some published studies suggest that these defence mechanisms and cellular-repair processes may themselves be impaired by such radiation (Hallberg and Johansson, 2004). As mentioned earlier, several epidemiological studies have found a relationship between time spent using mobile phones and an increased incidence of brain tumours (Hardell *et al.*, 2002; Lonn *et al.*, 2004).

This is not a matter of indulging in supposed conspiracies, as those hired to polish the public image of large companies and industries (often dubbed "merchants of doubt") would have us believe, but of keeping abreast of what is published in scientific journals—information that usually reaches the public filtered through whatever lens major media outlets choose to apply in each case. For it seems quite evident that the interests or preferences of major media organisations (often funded by powerful shareholders) do not necessarily coincide with those of society at large. This is a major public-health and environmental problem that has been ignored for several decades, since the widespread adoption of mobile phones. Regrettably, the media rarely address it—just as they rarely mention, with a few honourable exceptions, the serious effects of mRNA COVID vaccines (Patone *et al.*, 2022; Hwang *et al.*, 2025; Koizumi and Ono, 2025).

This is not the first time in recent history, nor will it be the last, that vested interests have concealed information of the utmost relevance for the public. Throughout the twentieth century, several episodes of "science hijacking" by major multinational corporations successfully delayed decision-making—as occurred in the cases of asbestos, tobacco, climate change, or GM crops (see review in Egilman and Böhme, 2005). The same may be happening with mobile-phone technology, as suggested by some specialised journals [2]. And when its effects are finally acknowledged, it is, unfortunately, often far too late for many people and, above all, for the environment, which bears the brunt—quietly and directly—of this dramatic delaying pattern characteristic of human economic and social realities.

The philosopher Jordi Pigem states in a recent article:

> *Wireless technologies today are surrounded by an aura of power, freedom and harmlessness not unlike the one that enveloped cigarettes half a century ago. If it can be shown that the telecommunications industry has 'conspired' (to paraphrase the 2006 court ruling on tobacco) to conceal the health damage caused by its devices, its downfall would be no less spectacular than that of the tobacco industry a few decades ago.*[3]

2 http://www.microwavenews.com/.

3 https://brownstoneesp.substack.com/p/humos-antenas-y-fraudes.

In that case, mobile phones would have to carry a warning about the risks of their use, just as cigarette packets do today.

On many occasions, there is great difficulty in experimentally demonstrating complex processes, and this obstacle is used as a reason — or an excuse — for scepticism, which maintains or favours business interests at the cost of postponing or burying scientific evidence. A typical problem in the scientific realm is the well-known fact that correlations cannot be used or adopted as proof of causation, as there may be other variables or circumstances not taken into account that could also be influencing the relationship observed between the variables studied.

The current chaotic situation should not lead to discouragement, but rather to the reactivation of the social movement that is fortunately re-emerging in towns and cities around the world in the face of this new and serious threat.

Owing to its parallels with the issues analysed in this book, we shall now turn to the powerful influence of the pharmaceutical industry on modern medicine. Clinical research, which shapes the way doctors practise medicine, is increasingly sponsored by the companies that manufacture medicines and medical devices. We are all aware of the importance of moderate exposure to sunlight, given its impact on vitamin D levels — a powerful ally of the immune system with significant effects on our overall health. Yet media campaigns warn only of its risks (melanoma), while simultaneously encouraging zero exposure and the use of sunscreens with ever-higher protection levels (sun-block filters) (Hallberg and Johansson, 2004). Meanwhile, paradoxically, studies are being published in major scientific journals reporting new discoveries and showing beneficial effects. For example, long-wave electromagnetic radiation from the sun penetrates more deeply into the body and enhances mitochondrial function, improving vision (Jeffery *et al.*, 2025).

One example of the conflict of interest within medicine is the industry-favouring bias found in studies funded by pharmaceutical companies. Several works carried out in recent years clearly reveal the reality of this dangerous bias (and we must not forget that health is one of people's most precious assets).

These systematic reviews have found that studies sponsored by the pharmaceutical industry are often more favourable to the sponsor's product compared with those funded by other sources, both in analyses of drug efficacy and in medical devices. A review of seventy-five studies showed that industry funding was associated with more frequent positive trial conclusions and statistically significant results (Lundh *et al.*, 2017). Sponsorship of studies on medicines and devices by pharmaceutical companies leads to more favourable results and conclusions regarding efficacy than those funded by other sources, such as public agencies. Another investigation concluded that systematic reviews with conflicts of interest related to pharmaceutical companies tend to reach conclusions favourable to industry and generally exhibit lower methodological quality than those without conflicts of interest (Hansen *et al.*, 2017).

Returning to the issue of electromagnetic radiation, one review examined whether the source of funding for research on the effects of low-intensity radiofrequency radiation introduces bias into the results. The authors found that studies funded by the telecommunications industry were significantly less likely to report adverse health effects compared with those funded by independent or governmental sources. This finding suggests the presence of funding bias — a well-documented phenomenon in other scientific fields — whereby economic interests may influence, consciously or unconsciously, research design, interpretation of findings, or selective publication. In the systematic review in question, studies of controlled exposure to radiofrequency radiation with health-related outcomes were analysed, including effects on electroencephalogram activity, cognitive or cardiovascular function, hormone levels, and subjective well-being. The authors found that studies funded exclusively by industry produced a greater number of results overall but showed a lower likelihood of reporting statistically significant effects compared with those funded by public agencies or charitable organisations. On the basis of these findings, they concluded that the interpretation of research on the health effects of radiofrequency radiation must take into account its source of funding (Huss *et al.*, 2006).

This conclusion reinforces what the American researcher Henry Lai, emeritus editor of *Electromagnetic Biology and Medicine*, had already pointed out years earlier: that industry-funded research is less likely to acknowledge the possible adverse effects of its products. According to Lai, this trend suggests a potential conflict of interest that may bias the production and dissemination of scientific knowledge in this field.

7.2 The Troublesome Role of the ICNIRP

In 2015, the association AVAATE produced a dossier on the ICNIRP (International Commission on Non-Ionizing Radiation Protection) in order to demonstrate the existence of numerous conflicts of interest among its members. Despite being a private body, the ICNIRP is recognised by the World Health Organization (WHO) as the reference entity for establishing the exposure limits to non-ionising radiation to which people (and other species) may be subjected so as to prevent such radiation from affecting their health. The fact that ICNIRP members incur various conflicts of interest — owing to their links with companies invested in the development of telecommunications and new technologies — undermines the impartiality that should govern the regulation of non-ionising radiation limits for the population. It is also difficult to understand why an international organisation such as the WHO, which has ample qualified public resources at its disposal to establish these limits appropriately, delegates to a private body matters that affect the public health of all humanity.[4]

Previously, AVAATE had prepared another report, which it sent to the European Ombudsman, requesting that the complaints concerning the situation of most members of the European working

4 http://www.avaate.org/spip.php?article2624.

group on electromagnetic waves — specifically regarding their proper objectivity — be examined and verified, and that the necessary initiatives be promoted to prevent the notorious and evident conflicts of interest involved.[5]

This same situation is occurring in many countries around the world. For example, the 2012 report of the Advisory Group on Non-Ionising Radiation (AGNIR) forms the basis of official advice on the safety of radiofrequency (RF) electromagnetic fields in the United Kingdom and draws on work carried out by health-protection agencies worldwide. This review contains incorrect and misleading statements, as well as omissions and conflicts of interest, which render it unsuitable for health-risk assessment. The executive summary and overall conclusions do not accurately reflect the available scientific evidence, nor do they adequately fulfil their responsibility to safeguard and protect citizens (Starkey, 2016).

It seems important to mention — as noted earlier — that major insurance companies have refused to cover possible health damage from mobile-phone masts, and that mobile phones increasingly include warnings (always in very small print, unreadable for the presbyopic), such as advising users to keep the device away from the head when initiating a call (as this is when it emits the most radiation).

In short, the industry is putting people's health at risk (Leal *et al.*, 2005) and generating environmental pollution which, unfortunately, is invisible and may have unpredictable effects on living beings.

7.3 International Scientific Appeals

In May 2015 an international scientific appeal was made public, signed by two hundred and seven researchers specialising in electromagnetic fields from forty different nations, warning that international protection guidelines for non-ionising EMFs (electromagnetic fields) are inadequate. The appeal stated that numerous recent

5 http://www.avaate.org/spip.php?article2577.

scientific publications have shown that EMFs affect living organisms at levels well below most international and national guidelines, and that the effects include increased cancer risk; cellular stress; elevated free-radical levels; genetic damage; structural and functional changes to the reproductive system; deficits in learning and memory; neurological disorders; and negative impacts on the general well-being of human beings. The harm goes beyond the human species, as there is growing evidence of detrimental effects on plants and animals.

These findings justify the call to the United Nations (UN) and to all Member States worldwide to urge the World Health Organization (WHO) to take a leading role in promoting the development of EMF guidelines that protect the population, to encourage precautionary measures, and to educate the general public about health risks—particularly for children and during the fetal developmental period. The appeal warns that, should no action be taken, the WHO would be failing in its mission as the international body responsible for safeguarding public health.

In 2017 this appeal was updated (the author of this book took part in it, signing it and providing the Spanish translation). The introduction stated:

> *International Appeal. Scientists Call for Protection from Non-Ionising Electromagnetic Field Exposure.*
>
> *We are scientists engaged in the study of the biological and health effects of non-ionising electromagnetic fields (EMFs). Based on research that has been peer-reviewed and published in scientific journals, we have serious concerns regarding the ubiquitous and increasing exposure to electromagnetic fields generated by electrical and wireless devices. These include — though are not limited to — radiofrequency-radiation (RFR) emitting devices such as mobile and cordless phones and their base stations, Wi-Fi, broadcasting antennas, smart meters and baby monitors, as well as electrical devices and infrastructure used for the supply of electricity that generate extremely low-frequency electromagnetic fields (ELF EMFs).*

By March 2018, the appeal had already been signed by two hundred and thirty-seven scientists specialising in electromagnetic fields and radiation from forty-one different nations.

More recently, two further international appeals have been launched. The first, promoted by Dr Hardell, an eminent Swedish researcher on the effects of mobile phones on the incidence of brain tumours, is addressed to the United Nations, the World Health Organization, and all governments. It urges them not to accept the ICNIRP guidelines, on the grounds that they are unscientific and pose a serious risk to human health and the environment, since they permit harmful exposure of the world's population, including the most vulnerable. These guidelines protect only industry, not public health, and therefore the appeal calls for the adoption of limits that genuinely protect against the known harmful effects of exposure to electromagnetic fields (with frequencies between 100 kHz and 300 GHz).

The second appeal, promoted by the American Arthur Firstenberg (who, sadly, has recently passed away) and signed by scientists, physicians, and environmental organisations, calls for a halt to the rollout of the 5G (fifth-generation) wireless network, including the 5G network of space satellites. Its message is unequivocal: the deployment of 5G is increasing exposure to radiofrequency (RF) radiation from telecommunications in comparison with 2G, 3G and 4G networks. Radiofrequency radiation has been shown to be harmful, and the deployment of 5G constitutes an experiment on humanity and the environment which, through the lens of international law, may be defined as a crime against humanity.

However, prior to these international appeals, many others had already been issued in various countries and regions in similar terms: Vienna (1998), Salzburg (2000), Alcalá (2001), the Freiburg Declaration (2002), Catania (2002), Benevento (2006), Brussels (2007), Venice (2008), the Netherlands (2009), Paris (2009), London (2009), Porto Alegre (2009), Copenhagen (2010) and Switzerland (2012), among others.

7.4 The Most Significant Research

There is no doubt about the need for continued research (although this must not be used as an excuse to delay the necessary measures once the evidence becomes overwhelming). Studies involving animals exposed to these forms of radiation can be highly revealing and essential for understanding the scale of the problem we are facing. As we have seen in previous sections of the book, beyond the other symptoms already described, one of the most debated and concerning issues is the possibility that such radiation may induce cancer.

Recently, the results of two major scientific studies—remarkable for their duration, cost, and importance—have been published and widely disseminated. The first was an American study carried out by the National Toxicology Program (NTP), with a cost of twenty-eight million dollars. The United States National Toxicology Program (NTP) is part of the National Institute of Environmental Health Sciences (NIEHS), itself a component of the National Institutes of Health (NIH) of the US Government. The research tested the two main types of modulation used in mobile telephony worldwide, GSM (2G) and UMTS (3G/4G), in a two-year rodent cancer bioassay under near-field exposure conditions. The experiments included additional assays to determine genotoxicity endpoints (Smith-Roe *et al.*, 2020). The results, published progressively in high-level scientific journals, showed clear evidence of carcinogenic activity and, more specifically, malignant schwannomas of the heart, malignant gliomas of the brain, and benign, malignant, or complex (combined) phaeochromocytomas of the adrenal medulla. They also found increased DNA damage (measured using the comet assay) in the frontal cortex of male mice, in the leukocytes of female mice, and in the hippocampus of male rats—indicating that mobile phone radiation may cause DNA damage and consequent carcinogenesis.

Professor James C. Lin, Chair of the ICNIRP Standing Committee on Physics and Technology from 2008 to 2012, and for many years editor of the leading scientific journal *Bioelectromagnetics*, published an article in the journal of the IEEE (the International Association of Engineers) discussing the NTP study results, noting that they suggest current radiofrequency exposure guidelines are inadequate to protect human health (Lin, 2019).

Professor Lin's article summarises the conclusions of a conference in which the fourteen scientists on the independent NTP peer-review panel agreed on this interpretation of the results. This independent review meeting on the National Toxicology Program study was held from 23 to 25 October 2017 at Research Triangle Park, North Carolina. During the meeting, the panel—composed of independent scientists with no representation of any institution, company, or governmental agency—evaluated the NTP research report on the genomic dose–response modelling approach. Until that point, Professor Lin had supported the opposing view, aligned with that of ICNIRP (International Commission on Non-Ionizing Radiation Protection), a private body that has for many years served as an adviser to the World Health Organization on this topic. As we have already explained, there is a longstanding record of direct or indirect support from the telecommunications industry to numerous ICNIRP members (a conflict of interest). It should therefore come as no surprise that Professor Lin is no longer a member of the exclusive ICNIRP group.

According to Dr Hardell, from the Department of Oncology at Örebro University (Sweden), who has led the group that has published the most research on this subject in high-impact scientific journals, the NTP's findings of schwannomas and gliomas in rodents are particularly concerning, as they corroborate the results reported by the human epidemiological studies conducted so far.

The second study was conducted in Italy over a ten-year period by the prestigious Ramazzini Institute and published in the scientific journal *Environmental Research* (Falcioni *et al.*, 2018). It is an extensive carcinogenicity study. The authors examined far-field exposure to 1800 MHz GSM EMF and reported results very similar to those of the NTP study described above. Specifically, they also found a higher incidence of brain and heart tumours in Sprague–Dawley rats exposed to mobile phone radiation. Their findings on far-field radiofrequency exposure (further from the radiation source) are consistent with and reinforce the NTP study's results on near-field exposure, as both found an increased incidence of brain and heart tumours in rodents exposed to radiofrequencies. Moreover, these tumours are of the same histological types as those observed in epidemiological studies involving human mobile phone users (Hardell *et al.*, 2007). Both experimental studies provide sufficient evidence to call for a re-evaluation of the conclusions reached by the International Agency for Research on Cancer (IARC) of the World Health Organization regarding the carcinogenic potential of radiofrequencies in humans.

Kostoff *et al.* (2020) emphasise that most laboratory experiments conducted to date were not designed to detect the most serious adverse effects reflecting the real-world environment in which wireless radiation systems operate, since many experiments do not include the pulsing and modulation of the carrier signal, and most do not account for the synergistic adverse effects of other toxic stimuli.

8

FORETELLING EARTHQUAKES

The earliest known reference to unusual animal behaviour prior to an earthquake comes from ancient Greece, specifically the fourth century BC (Schaal, 1988). According to historical accounts, rats, weasels, snakes and centipedes abandoned their burrows and moved to safer areas several days before the arrival of a destructive earthquake. There is abundant anecdotal evidence of animals (fish, amphibians, reptiles, birds, mammals and insects) displaying strange behaviour from several weeks to mere seconds before a seismic event. However, until very recently the biophysical mechanism that could explain this phenomenon had remained unresolved.

The countries that have shown the greatest scientific interest in this subject are China and Japan, and this is no coincidence, for Japan is one of the most earthquake-prone nations in the world. Situated close to a major tectonic subduction zone, it has suffered devastating earthquakes that have claimed countless lives and caused immense damage. Researchers have long studied animal behaviour in the hope of discovering what creatures might hear or sense before the Earth shakes, and of harnessing this particular sensitivity as a predictive tool.

8.1 Key Factors Underlying Perception

There is an explanation for animals' ability to detect earthquakes a few seconds before they occur, well before humans are able to perceive them. The seismic waves generated during earthquakes fall into two broad categories: P-waves and S-waves.

In P-waves, also known as primary or compressional waves, the particles transmitting the pressure waveform move in the same direction as the wave's propagation. These oscillatory movements travel faster and therefore arrive earlier than S-waves, or secondary waves, in which the particles move perpendicular to the direction of propagation.

Humans can perceive S-waves; however, we are unable to detect P-waves. By contrast, many animals can sense P-waves because their sensory capacities are more highly developed. This would explain their earlier perception—only a few seconds before the quake—and therefore why they react before humans become aware of what is happening (Lakshmi *et al.*, 2014).

However, the ability of certain animals to predict seismic activity days or even weeks in advance is far more difficult to explain. One theory suggesting that animals exhibit "predictive" behaviour prior to an earthquake relates to missing household pets (Schaal, 1988). A study conducted in the San Francisco Bay Area found an increase in local newspaper advertisements reporting missing pets prior to several earthquakes, although a later analysis did not uncover any genuine correlation (Lakshmi *et al.*, 2014).

A study carried out at Osaka University (Japan), in which the circadian rhythms of mice were recorded, showed unusual behaviour before the earthquake that struck the Kobe region on 17 January 1995. Locomotor activity on the previous day (16 January) increased dramatically, several times above the standard deviation, which was interpreted as an indication that the mice perceived some sort of pre-seismic cues (Yokoi *et al.*, 2003).

During the Wenchuan (China) earthquake of magnitude 8.0 on 12 May 2008, the locomotor activity and circadian rhythm of eight mice were monitored over a period of thirty-eight days. Researchers found that six of the animals experienced a drastic decrease in mobility three days before the earthquake, accompanied by a loss of circadian rhythm. This behavioural change lasted six days, after which their locomotor activity returned to its original state (Li *et al.*, 2009).

It has also been suggested that some people may show a degree of sensitivity—such as headaches—prior to earthquakes, although there is considerable scientific scepticism regarding this claim (Kirschvink, 2000). Indeed, certain individuals report experiencing an unpleasant pressure or headache that lasts for weeks and then suddenly disappears moments before the quake (Lakshmi *et al.*, 2014).

The unusual behaviour of animals also gives rise to considerable controversy within the scientific community. Although there have been documented cases of strange animal behaviour prior to earthquakes, the view of the United States Geological Survey – a government agency that provides scientific information about the Earth – is that no reproducible connection has ever been found between any specific behaviour and the occurrence of an earthquake. According to American seismologists, most of the existing data are based on anecdotal, retrospective recollections referring to a very short period immediately preceding such events. They argue that the widespread belief that animals can anticipate earthquakes is not yet sufficiently supported by scientific evidence, and there remains substantial scepticism regarding this possibility.

However, in a highly significant study published in 2010 and conducted in L'Aquila, the capital of the Abruzzo region in central Italy, researchers monitored the reproductive activity of a population of common toads (*Bufo bufo*) before, during and after an earthquake. The toads, located 75 km from the epicentre, displayed a dramatic change in behaviour five days before the quake, abandoning their reproductive activity and not resuming normal behaviour until several days after the seismic event. The type of pre-earthquake environmental stimulus to which the toads responded remains unknown, but the cessation of their reproductive behaviour coincided with preseismic disturbances in the ionosphere, phenomena typically associated with tectonic movements and detectable through the generation of very low frequency (VLF) radio waves (Grant & Halliday, 2010).

There are numerous anecdotal accounts of reptiles waking abruptly, amphibians fleeing or deep-sea fish rising to the surface; yet given that major earthquakes are extremely rare and unpredictable, the events surrounding them are almost impossible to study in detail. In this respect, the case of the L'Aquila toads was different, as Rachel Grant, the author of the study, had been monitoring the colony as part of her doctoral research. She observed the abrupt disappearance of the ninety-six toads that had been breeding there, with almost none remaining within three days, and with no meteorological or other environmental changes to account for it. Apparently, following the publication of the study, NASA expressed interest in the findings and contacted Dr Grant.

Scientists at the United States space agency have been studying the physicochemical changes that occur when rocks are subjected to intense pressure and stress, and are considering whether these variations might be related to the mass exodus of the toads—perhaps linked to potential alterations in groundwater chemistry prior to seismic events (Grant *et al.*, 2011).

During the build-up to earthquakes, geophysical processes unfold across different spatial and temporal scales within the Earth's crust, on its surface and even in the ionosphere, and these processes also affect living organisms. In 2011, a study was carried out involving several interdisciplinary researchers—biologists, geologists and physicists from various British and Brazilian universities, as well as NASA—in Yanachaga National Park in Peru. The abundance of mammals and birds was recorded over a thirty-day period using motion-triggered camera traps before the magnitude-7 Contamana earthquake, which struck on 24 August 2011. In addition, ionospheric disturbances derived from nocturnal very low frequency (VLF) waves were monitored. Animal activity was found to decrease significantly during the three weeks preceding the earthquake, compared with periods of low seismic activity. For their part, the ionospheric disturbances began two weeks before the quake.

The concurrence of these two observations—of phenomena that are highly different and seemingly unconnected—as potential precursors or predictors of the tremor is of great interest, because it has recently been proposed that the multitude of pre-earthquake phenomena observed may all be driven by a single underlying physical process (Grant *et al.*, 2015).

In a study conducted in Indonesia on African catfish (*Clarias gariepinus*) kept in aquaria, a marked increase in activity was observed in the five specimens shortly before the arrival of an earthquake, despite the fish having shown very little activity for more than a month. The authors suggest that this behavioural change may indicate an ability to detect increased preseismic activity, possibly in response to the rise in electromagnetic waves that precede earthquakes (Ferasyi *et al.*, 2013).

A review published by researchers in India summarises global studies on earthquake prediction based on animal behaviour. This line of research is grounded in the superior ability of animals, compared with humans, to perceive certain geophysical stimuli that typically precede seismic events (Bhargava *et al.*, 2009).

The Republic of China has established an operational earthquake-prediction network across several provinces. In 1968, it set up the first experimental station for predicting earthquakes through biological observation in Hsingtai Province, and others were later created. In August 1971, the country's State Seismological Bureau began collecting reports of unusual animal behaviour for this purpose. Four years later, drawing on these observations as well as geophysical measurements, it successfully evacuated the city of Haicheng several hours before the magnitude 7.3 earthquake that struck on 4 February 1975. The most striking observation was that snakes emerged to the surface in the middle of winter—only to freeze thereafter—when under normal circumstances these reptiles hibernate throughout the winter period (Wang *et al.*, 2006). During the first three days of February, there were also reports of odd behaviour in cows, horses, dogs and pigs. This earthquake caused considerable damage to buildings and farmland, and it is estimated that the evacuation may have saved more than one hundred thousand lives.

Similarly, there were reports of anomalous animal behaviour prior to the magnitude 8.2 Tangshan earthquake in 1976, but unlike the previous case, no warning was issued, with the devastating result of around 240,000 fatalities. It appears that not all earthquakes are preceded by unusual animal behaviour, and only through research will it be possible to identify the biogeophysical factors that distinguish one event from another.

Many animals escaped the great tsunami that struck Asia in 2004. Elephants in Sri Lanka and Sumatra moved to higher ground before the gigantic wave reached the shore, sweeping everything in its path. In Thailand, a herd of buffalo was grazing on the beach when they suddenly raised their heads and looked towards the sea, ears pricked. They then turned and headed for the hillside, followed by bewildered villagers—who in doing so saved their lives. There are similar accounts of dog owners perplexed because their pets refused to go on their usual morning walk along the beach (Sheldrake, 2005).

> A wide range of vertebrates display "early-warning" behaviours that we already understand in relation to other types of events, so it is possible that an escape response to an earthquake may have evolved from this pre-existing genetic predisposition. An instinctive reaction following a P-wave, seconds before a larger S-wave, is not a "great leap", so to speak. But what about other precursors that may occur days or weeks before an earthquake and which we do not yet understand? If, indeed, there are precursors to a significant earthquake that remain to be identified—such as ground tilting, changes in groundwater, or electrical or magnetic variations—then it is conceivable that some animals may be able to detect these signals and associate their perception with an imminent earthquake.[6]

6 (Kirschvink, 2000).

Precisely these factors do exist, and we shall examine them in the following section.

8.2 The Elusive Factors

Several studies conducted in the former USSR suggest that, immediately before earthquakes, broadband electromagnetic radiation is generated across a wide range of frequencies. To record this phenomenon, an experiment was carried out in 1980 at the United States Space Research Observatory in Japan, as part of the USSR–Japan Cooperation Programme. The intensity of waves recorded at a frequency of 81 kHz remained relatively low throughout the day. However, roughly half an hour before the earthquake that occurred on 31 March 1980, the instrument registered an anomalous increase in the intensity of these waves. Moreover, similar 81 kHz emissions were observed prior to the magnitude-5 and magnitude-6 earthquakes of 25 September 1980 and 28 January 1981. VLF wave data recorded synoptically in Sugadaira (Japan) suggest that pulsed radiation at frequencies below 1.5 kHz also occurred shortly before the quake (Gokhberg *et al.*, 1982).

Marsha Adams, an independent researcher in San Francisco who studies earthquakes, claims to have developed sensors that measure low-frequency electromagnetic signals, enabling her to predict earthquakes with more than 90% accuracy. Adams suspects that the low-frequency electromagnetic signals generated by the fracturing of crystalline rocks deep within the Earth along fault lines are biologically active and constitute the very signals detected by animals possessing this sensory capability (Lakshmi *et al.*, 2014).

As we have already seen, animals with highly developed navigational systems are particularly sensitive to electromagnetic fields. Birds, for instance, possess a highly sophisticated orientation system and respond markedly to changes in atmospheric conditions. Both they and other animals display anomalous behaviours during events such as solar eclipses, showing reactions ranging from lethargy to restlessness. Various studies attribute these responses to the influence of electromagnetic waves. As we explained in Chapter 4, ionisation in the ionosphere is lower at night, allowing electromagnetic waves to propagate up to a hundred times more effectively across the Earth's surface; this effect of unexpected incoming electromagnetic impulses could also explain the early-warning system that animals appear to possess for predicting earthquakes (Warnke, 2007).

We have recently proposed a biogeophysical mechanism that bears strong similarities to, and is entirely compatible with, the atmospheric *sferics* hypothesis put forward by Panagopoulos and Balmori (2017), discussed in detail in Chapter 3. It concerns the possible interrelationship between the electromagnetic precursor radiations of earthquakes—which would act as a stimulus—and the anomalous behaviour displayed by animals prior to seismic events. The low-frequency, low-intensity seismic electrical signals generated in the prefocal area several days before an earthquake satisfy all the conditions established for an explanatory model of these bioeffects (Dologlou, 2010).

That author suggests that the anomalous behaviour of the toads described earlier, observed before the 2009 L'Aquila earthquake (Grant & Halliday, 2010), may have been caused by processes related to the activity of the seismic electrical signals developed in the prefocal region. This argument is supported by two key points: first, the electrical signals meet all the conditions set out in the bioeffects model of Panagopoulos *et al.* (2000), namely a low-frequency, low-intensity electric field; and, secondly, they are emitted from the preseismic area where the unusual toad behaviour was observed (Dologlou, 2010).

In our study, published in the prestigious scientific journal *STOTEN* (Panagopoulos *et al.*, 2020), we explain that, days or even weeks before major earthquakes, changes in animal behaviour are observed at distances of up to 500 km from the seismic epicentre. Simultaneously, seismic electric signals (SES) and geomagnetic and ionospheric disturbances are detected at similar distances. SES consist of individual unipolar pulses and/or groups of such pulses, with an average inter-pulse frequency on the order of ~0.01 Hz and an electric field intensity on the order of ~10^{-5}–10^{-4} V/m. In that study, we demonstrated that living organisms can detect SES activity through the biophysical mechanism proposed for the action of electromagnetic fields (EMFs) on cells—the forced-oscillation mechanism of ions—according to which polarised EMFs can cause irregular activation of electrosensitive ion channels in cell membranes, thereby disrupting the cell's electrochemical balance.

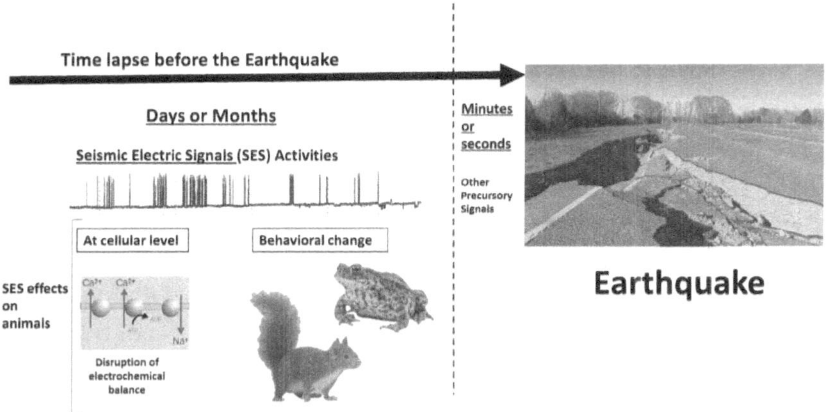

Figure 27: Explanation of animals' early detection of earthquakes, according to Panagopoulos et al., 2020.

Furthermore, ion-channel dysfunction alters intracellular ion concentrations, triggering the overproduction of reactive oxygen species (highly *reactive oxygen-containing* molecules known as ROS), which can damage biomolecules (including DNA) and cause oxidative stress through the cellular systems and enzymes that generate them, such as the mitochondrial electron transport chain, NADPH/NADH oxidase systems, nitric oxide synthases (NOS), and others.

Therefore, geomagnetic and ionospheric disturbances may be perceived via this mechanism, the same one that explains meteoropathy—that is, the ability of sensitive individuals to perceive the approach of thunderstorms through the action of *sferics* (Panagopoulos

& Balmori, 2017). Consequently, the centuries-old anecdotal reports of animals sensing intense earthquakes and exhibiting unusual behaviour, more recently documented by systematic studies, can now be explained for the first time on the basis of the electromagnetic nature of all living organisms and the electromagnetic signals emitted prior to earthquakes (SES).

In addition, this process constitutes an integrated mechanism that explains all known adverse biological and health effects documented as being induced by anthropogenic electromagnetic fields (Panagopoulos *et al.*, 2000, 2015, 2025) (see also Section 3.3).

During the major earthquake that struck Minahasa, Indonesia, Indian researchers observed and analysed very low frequency (VLF) electromagnetic signals preceding the seismic event, recorded at frequencies of 5, 7, 9 and 12 kHz. These signals were detected on 16 November 2008 in Kolkata (India) using specialised receivers. Peaks in signal variation began to appear several days before the earthquake and continued for several days afterwards, gradually diminishing until they disappeared. The temporal variability of natural electromagnetic signals in the VLF band overlaps with the preseismic records (De *et al.*, 2011). Given their similarity to the *sferics* generated in the atmosphere discussed earlier (Chapter 3), these authors also refer to the electromagnetic radiations accompanying seismic movements as *sferics*, while clearly differentiating them from atmospheric ones.

According to Japanese researchers, an objective method for identifying electromagnetic signals associated with an earthquake at a given location is to verify that they coincide temporally with the seismic event and originate predominantly from a specific direction, such as the epicentre or the focal area of the quake. In contrast, *sferics* generated by atmospheric discharges (lightning) have a much more dispersed geographical origin, reflecting the broad and spatially variable distribution of storms (Asada *et al.*, 2001). The electromagnetic signals in the 1–10 kHz frequency range associated with earthquakes are pulsed and also polarised—an essential feature from the standpoint of their biological activity (Panagopoulos *et al.*, 2015), as discussed in Chapter 3. After investigating four different earthquakes, Asada and colleagues (2001) demonstrated that the electromagnetic signals generated are not confined to the precise moment of the quake; rather, the maximum activity of VLF electromagnetic radiation occurs between one and four days before the seismic event.

As we have seen in previous chapters, this type of polarised electromagnetic pulses is perceived by a wide range of species and sensitive individuals, which can fully explain the observations regarding early warning behaviour or predictive responses displayed by many different groups of animals, as documented in the scientific literature.

Another group of Japanese researchers went a step further by conducting experiments in which granite, basalt, and marble rocks were subjected to high pressure using a 500-ton compression machine. The aim was to detect both acoustic waves and the electromagnetic radiation generated, in an attempt to reproduce the unusual animal behaviour observed prior to major earthquakes. As a result, the researchers observed atypical animal behaviour during the compression experiments, with simultaneous detection of pulsed electromagnetic waves, preceding the detection of the sound waves (electromagnetic radiation travels far faster than sound waves). Furthermore, to avoid potential subjective factors in the observation of animal behaviour, the researchers quantified hypothalamic neurotransmitters—adrenaline, noradrenaline, and serotonin—in the blood plasma of the experimental rats, before and after the rock fractures. They observed an increase in noradrenaline and a decrease in adrenaline, a response differing from reactions to other stressors but similar to that caused by exposure to pulsed electromagnetic waves. For this reason, they concluded that the anomalous behaviour of animals observed prior to earthquakes is fundamentally caused by the pulsed electromagnetic waves naturally generated during seismic processes (Ikeya *et al.*, 2000).

Moreover, it has long been known in the scientific community that atmospheric activity can change in the period preceding earthquakes. The generation of electromagnetic phenomena across various frequency ranges, covering the ELF to VHF bands, has been recorded by several independent research groups in relation to the Kobe earthquake, which occurred on 17 January 1995 and reached a magnitude of 7.2. On 9 and 10 January, strong preseismic electromagnetic wave peaks were observed, presumably originating from the earthquake's focal area. However, the researchers could not distinguish whether these observations were related to the earthquake or to atmospheric discharges from storms, as lightning activity also peaked on those same days. The anomalies increased as the catastrophe approached, consistent with many reports of unusual interference in radio and television transmissions. Anomalous propagation of artificial electromagnetic waves in the VLF and VHF ranges was detected, suggesting that the ionosphere might also experience disturbances during the final stage of earthquake preparation (Nagao *et al.*, 2002).

Researchers in Taiwan demonstrated, using a network of lightning detectors that monitored continuously from fifteen days before to fifteen days after the Chi-Chi earthquake (China), that lightning generation increased significantly four days prior to the seismic event, and that anomalies in the ionosphere and atmosphere were electromagnetically coupled with the earthquake (Tsai *et al.*, 2006). These findings indicate that there is an electromagnetic connection between seismic processes and anomalies in the atmosphere and ionosphere. Indeed, as we will see in the next chapter, when radiation from outer space is also taken into account, the problem becomes even more complex

9

THE EARTH'S GEOMAGNETIC ACTIVITY AND SOLAR RADIATION

Up to this point, we have mainly examined the capacity of *sferics*—both those of atmospheric origin and those generated by earthquakes—to trigger biological and health-related effects in living organisms. However, there are other factors that further complicate the picture of natural low-frequency electromagnetic radiation.

When the influx of high-energy particles from the Sun (the solar wind) becomes particularly intense and prolonged, to the extent that it modifies the characteristics of the upper layers of the atmosphere, geomagnetic storms arise. These solar storms usually last between one and five days, after which normal magnetic conditions are restored (Palmer *et al.*, 2006).

The possibility that such solar eruptions might affect human health at ground level has been debated for several decades. The growing number of articles published in recent years highlights the significant influence of these geophysical factors—changes in solar activity and the associated geomagnetic disturbances—on physiological, biological and health parameters in healthy individuals. Although objective difficulties remain, research in this field is extremely valuable for protecting humans from their harmful effects (Stoilova & Dimitrova, 2008). Geomagnetic disturbances may also influence work efficiency, concentration and levels of anxiety. This underscores the relevance of the relationship between outer space and human physiology, not only for the prevention or treatment of certain physical and psychological disorders, but also for the overall improvement of human wellbeing (Papiliou *et al.*, 2011).

A team of British and French researchers published a review of studies conducted in the field of heliobiology, the branch of science concerned with the impact of solar activity on living organisms—particularly humans—as well as the various causal mechanisms involved (Palmer *et al.*, 2006). It has been shown that extremely high or low values of geomagnetic activity—i.e. significant deviations from normal levels for a given latitude—may give rise to health problems in living beings. Moreover, it is estimated that between 10 and 15% of the population is predisposed to experiencing adverse health effects as a result of such geomagnetic variations (Palmer *et al.*, 2006). Research findings on the influence of geomagnetic activity on human physiological parameters are unequivocal: human health can be affected by solar activity and the associated geophysical disturbances (Papiliou *et al.*, 2011). As can be seen, there are similarities that echo phenomena such as electrosensitivity and meteoropathy, which affect a specific proportion of the population, as noted in earlier chapters of this book.

Wild species are also affected. As discussed in Section 6.4, geomagnetic field alterations occur during solar storms, and these have been linked to an increase in grey whale strandings (Granger *et al.*, 2020). Most researchers studying the relationship between solar radiation and the biosphere agree that the Sun's effect on living organisms is predominantly electromagnetic in nature (Khabarova & Dimitrova, 2008). Variations in solar activity, geomagnetic activity, and the concentrations of ions and electrons in the ionosphere are closely correlated and interconnected through complex geophysical processes. This interdependence makes it difficult to identify in isolation the key natural environmental factors responsible for the observed biological and physical effects. It has been proposed that many of these effects may be mediated through alterations in the Schumann resonance signal, a mechanism through which all these phenomena would be interrelated (Cherry, 2002).

It is, moreover, considered unlikely that a single biological mechanism could account for all the phenomena observed and described. Nevertheless, several widely recognised processes have been linked to exposure to low-frequency radiation and pulses. These include altered melatonin release induced by the action of radiation on the pineal gland; changes in cellular permeability through effects on ion channels; and the modification of brain waves as a result of external electromagnetic interference. All of these mechanisms have also been discussed in earlier chapters.

The scientific literature has repeatedly documented a direct relationship between terrestrial magnetic disturbances and the dynamics of myocardial infarction. Experimental studies show a significant increase in the rate of heart attacks during episodes of strong geomagnetic disturbances (Villoresi *et al.*, 1998). In this regard, a study published in the prestigious journal *Nature* found a high correlation between the monthly average of daily hospital admissions for heart attacks and the Earth's geomagnetic activity (Malin & Srivastava, 1979).

These findings are not isolated. Subsequent research has revealed considerable increases in mean systolic and diastolic blood pressure values coinciding with rises in geomagnetic activity. In particular, blood pressure values have been observed to rise approximately two days before a geomagnetic storm and to remain elevated until two days after the event (Dimitrova *et al.*, 2009).

Between 1994 and 2002, a study was conducted in which 4,018 Slovak aircrew members aged between eighteen and sixty— all in good health—underwent medical examinations. The investigation covered periods of heightened solar and geomagnetic activity, with particular emphasis on measuring mean systolic and diastolic blood pressure values (Papiliou *et al.*, 2011). The study analysed the statistical significance of the relationship between daily variations in geomagnetic indices—indicators of terrestrial geomagnetic activity—and the blood pressure parameters mentioned. The results showed a significant correlation, leading to the conclusion that geomagnetic disturbances are indeed related to changes in human physiological parameters.

Various studies suggest that responses to geomagnetic disturbances vary according to sex, with women generally being more sensitive to geomagnetic fields than men (Khabarova & Dimitrova, 2008). Likewise, individuals with arterial hypertension represent the group most vulnerable to the effects of geomagnetic storms, whereas those with hypotension appear to be less susceptible. With respect to age, the group most affected comprises people over sixty-five, who display greater vulnerability both in blood pressure levels and in the incidence of myocardial infarction, the latter tending to increase in the days preceding and following geomagnetic disturbances (Mendoza & Peña, 2010).

As noted earlier, it has been proposed that the geomagnetic anomalies occurring prior to earthquakes may also partly explain the capacity of certain animals to perceive and anticipate such events, particularly those possessing a well-developed magnetoreception system for navigational purposes (Kirschvink, 2000).

Geomagnetic disturbances have also been linked to a reduction in the excretion of a melatonin metabolite (Burch *et al.*, 1999), indicating that they exert a direct effect on the activity of the pineal gland, which is responsible for producing this important hormone, a key regulator of circadian rhythms and several other highly relevant physiological processes.

Experimental studies carried out in Azerbaijan, aimed at investigating the potential effects of variability in solar, geomagnetic and cosmic radiation on different biological systems—particularly the human brain, general health and psycho-emotional state—have shown that intense episodes of electromagnetic activity can induce significant alterations in cerebral bioelectrical activity. These changes are associated with marked emotional effects and notable autonomic manifestations in the individuals exposed (Babayev & Allahverdiyeva, 2007).

A number of investigations have identified a correlation between terrestrial magnetic activity and the average number of recorded deaths (Warnke, 2007). Among the adverse effects on mental health, one of the most widely studied has been depression, a condition that in some cases may lead to suicidal behaviour (Palmer *et al.*, 2006). In this regard, South African and Australian researchers conducted a retrospective study spanning thirteen years, using official data on geomagnetic storms and recorded suicides in South Africa. The results revealed a significant correlation between geomagnetic activity and suicide incidence, confirming previous findings regarding the influence of environmental magnetic fields on human behaviour (Gordon & Berk, 2003). The same researchers later drew similar conclusions from an analysis of data from Australia (Berk *et al.*, 2006).

Research has also been undertaken that jointly evaluates geomagnetic and solar indices alongside various climatic factors, including six meteorological parameters. The results indicate that the combination of these factors generates correlation levels that exceed those observed when each parameter is analysed separately (Khabarova & Dimitrova, 2008). This finding suggests an overlap of biological effects derived from different causes—solar, geomagnetic and meteorological.

In Lithuania, a study was conducted that examined hospital admissions for approximately two thousand patients in relation to solar and geomagnetic activity, also taking into account meteorological variables at the time of admission. The results confirmed that in patients with a history of infarction, angina pectoris, or pulmonary or renal disease, exposure to solar radiation increased the number of hospital admissions by 50% (Vencloviene *et al.*, 2013). It is particularly noteworthy that in patients with pre-existing renal disease the risk rises markedly when geomagnetic disturbances coincide with episodes of low atmospheric pressure in the troposphere. As noted in earlier chapters, low-pressure systems tend to be associated with the arrival of cold fronts and the generation of atmospheric storms and *sferics*.

As a general conclusion from what has been examined thus far, we can state that in a stable geomagnetic environment, low-frequency electromagnetic pulses originating in the atmosphere (known as *sferics*) are primarily regulated by meteorological factors, especially cold fronts. However, during periods of intense solar activity, or due to other factors that alter the Earth's geomagnetic characteristics—such as earthquakes or cosmic radiation—there is a superposition of electromagnetic effects from these various sources, which impact living beings in a combined manner. In addition, when interpreting results and assessing their potential biological effects, it is essential to consider other potential co-factors, such as the presence of artificial or anthropogenic electromagnetic pollution (Palmer *et al.*, 2006).

9.1 New Threats to the Atmosphere

The launch of hundreds of satellites for commercial purposes represents a new threat to ecosystems. It leads to a deterioration in astronomical observation and in the experience of the night sky; it increases space debris, and it may even interfere with animal orientation—both through changes in visible bright objects and through the rise in radio-frequency emissions.

In recent years, many enthusiasts of night-sky observation—as well as casual passers-by—have had the chance to witness a new and previously unseen spectacle in the firmament. A distinct trail, reminiscent of a comet's tail, would rise slowly in the western sky, gradually breaking apart into a train of several dozen luminous points that drifted away from one another until they vanished into the night. Although many people may have assumed that they were observing a natural phenomenon, such as a bolide, meteor or "shooting star", the reality is quite different. In the orbital space surrounding the Earth, environmental problems are worsening rapidly due to the increasing number of anthropogenic space objects, including the new satellite constellations (such as SpaceX Starlink, each typical launch of which places between forty and sixty satellites into orbit (Figure 28).

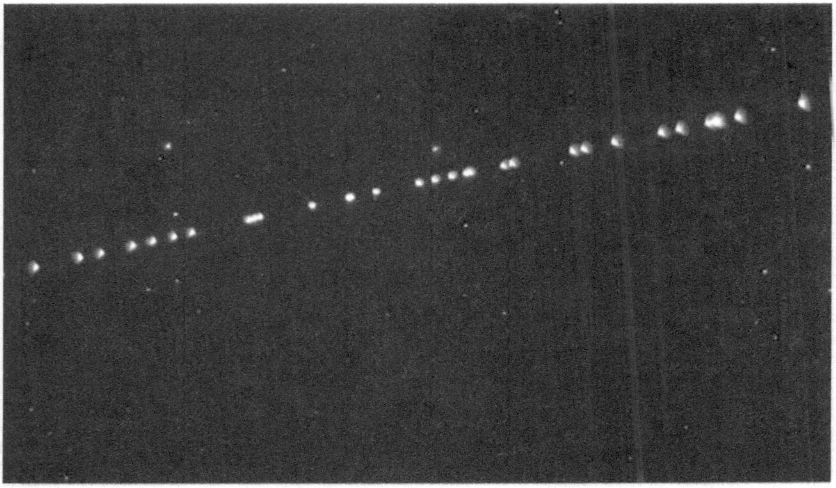

Figure 28: A typical train of SpaceX Starlink satellites following launch.

For this reason, in April 2022, the journal *Nature Astronomy* published an important article by a broad group of astronomers from research centres in the United Kingdom, the United States, Germany, Canada and the Netherlands. These researchers of the universe call for the orbital space around the Earth (roughly between 80–100 and 36,000 kilometres in altitude) to be regarded as an ecosystem in its own right, subject to the same care, concerns and general regulations as the oceans and the atmosphere, with which it shares common environmental problems (Lawrence *et al.*, 2022). To this end, they propose that this layer should be legally considered a global commons, since the growing commercial exploitation of what may at first sight appear to be an unlimited and freely available resource is, in reality, externalising its true costs. In view of the increasing private uses of outer space, they warn of the need to consider the damage being caused to professional astronomy, to star observation and to the cultural significance of the sky.

9.1.1 Interference with Space Telescopes

As far as optical astronomy is concerned, some telescopes have already experienced an increase in images affected by streaks, rising from 0.5% at the end of 2019 to 18% in August 2021. Radio telescopes are also affected by artificial satellites, which use radio signals to transmit data back and forth between ground stations and end-user antennas. The major issue lies in detecting faint celestial objects against this anthropogenic background, since emissions from satellites can be far stronger than the astronomical objects being sought. A useful analogy would be trying to listen to very quiet music in an excessively noisy room. Unlike the situation with optical images, the effect on radio telescopes is not a streak across the field but a complex impact across the entire image, which may be difficult to recognise and remove.

The Hubble Space Telescope is located in the Earth's closest orbital region (100–2,000 km), and occasionally a satellite can produce an extremely bright streak that erases a significant fraction of the image. Between 2% and 8% of this telescope's images have been affected by satellite streaks, and it has been shown that the frequency is increasing over time. At the current rate of launches of new satellite constellations, it is estimated that by the end of this decade one third of Hubble's images will be affected.

9.1.2 Impact on the Night Sky

The sky also holds significant cultural importance and has inspired deeply rooted traditions across the world since the dawn of human history, such as annual chronologies and star-based navigation among some Indigenous peoples. Access to an unpolluted night-sky environment that allows for the enjoyment and contemplation of the firmament—including unobstructed views of the stars—should be regarded as a right for all people. A much larger number of artificial satellites can significantly alter our entire perception of the night sky, appearing as "false stars".

9.1.3 Space Debris

An unprecedented growth in space debris is under way, consisting of abandoned satellite remnants, rocket stages, and fragments resulting from break-ups, explosions and collisions. If avoidance measures are not implemented, the current density of debris implies that, on average, there will be one collision per satellite every fifty years in the lowest orbits involving an object of 10 cm or larger.

In addition, all rocket launches generate emissions with negative impacts on the atmosphere, including CO_2, NO_x, soot and H_2O in the mesosphere. Until now, these have been minor contributors to global pollution, but the large number of launches required to build and maintain constellations of thousands of satellites could substantially increase their impact.

9.1.4 Effects on Terrestrial Ecosystems

Numerous animal species—from insects to mammals and birds—orient themselves during their migratory movements using several complementary navigation systems, among which the stars and the Milky Way play a role. It is estimated that approximately 40% of bird species migrate, and around 80% travel at night, many of them relying on the stars for navigation. Although we cannot yet know whether these species will be sensitive to these new additional points of light, which appear to move rapidly across the sky, reasonable predictions of potentially significant harm are already appearing in the scientific literature.

Furthermore, satellites communicate with ground stations using radio signals (radio frequencies). Satellite constellations emit radio frequencies that, although at low levels, can reach the Earth, adding to those already emitted by the millions of telecommunications antennas constructed worldwide over the past twenty-five years. For this reason, electromagnetic pollution has increased exponentially across the globe in recent years.

As we have seen throughout the book, human-made electromagnetic fields can produce harmful effects on people, animals and plants. Their potential impacts have been identified as an important emerging issue for global conservation and biological diversity (Sutherland *et al.*, 2019). Recent findings also indicate interference from anthropogenic radio frequencies with the orientation systems of animals. Consequently, it has been proposed that this saturation of space with anthropogenic radio frequencies carries an unpredictable risk of undesirable biological consequences for different animal groups.

Like all other ecosystems, orbital space has a limited carrying capacity. This limit has not yet been defined, but it seems evident that if it is used freely without a joint management system, this orbital carrying capacity is likely to become saturated, hampering safe activity in space operations, among other problems. For all the reasons discussed, high-level decision-makers must take into account the environmental impact of satellite constellations—including their launch, operation and subsequent debris—and foster a willingness among all stakeholders to create an ethical, sustainable and shared use of orbital space.

10

WE ARE PART OF NATURE

In ancient and early primitive cultures, the essential elements of nature were venerated, and human beings felt themselves to be part of the natural world. There existed a sense of identification between humans and nature that led them to worship mountains, forests or the sun with a religious, magical or mythical sentiment.

From the Renaissance onwards, however, the rise of the sciences and the increasing interest in understanding the natural world brought about a gradual distancing from it, and even a sense of opposition, as nature came to be conceived as a material object, open to domination and transformation. In the centuries that followed, humanity persisted in its attempts to master the forces of nature through science and technology, fostering a sense of power rather than protection.

With the arrival of the twentieth century, and the growing emergence of serious environmental problems — such as the depletion of natural resources, the energy crisis, climate change, and the pollution of air, water and soil, together with waste accumulation and the rapid loss of biodiversity — humanity once again became aware of its profound connection with the natural world. This situation compelled societies to adopt attitudes of concern and respect, as well as a more integrated vision of the human being within the natural environment, leaving behind the anthropocentrism that had characterised previous centuries.

The appearance of the studies and conclusions of the Club of Rome, the rise of environmental groups and the Green movement, the United Nations Conference on the Human Environment, and the Brundtland Report on "our common future" set the guidelines for what is now known as "sustainable development". Even today, this remains a somewhat utopian goal: an aspiration involving responsible behaviour and good intentions, yet difficult for humanity to fully assume and achieve.

More than a century and a half ago, Charles Darwin demonstrated that human beings — who regard themselves as very different from and generally superior to the thousands of species inhabiting planet Earth — are, in fact, fundamentally similar to all the others. We are the result of a changing process through time, in which some species emerge while others disappear, each descending from earlier forms through natural selection and following distinct adaptive pathways.

Humans are probably incomparably superior in terms of intelligence, yet we will never possess hearing as acute as that of nocturnal birds of prey, eyesight as sharp as that of diurnal raptors, or a sense of smell as developed as that of predatory carnivores. Nor will we ever perceive the electromagnetic signals of the environment with the sensitivity of bees. This means we are superior in some aspects — unquestionably important ones, such as intelligence and thought — but there are sensory abilities and capacities in countless other species that we barely understand. What use is the lateral line to fish? What purpose does Jacobson's organ serve in snakes? What abilities have bats developed to navigate using ultrasound (echolocation)? How do salmon, prior to spawning, return with such precision to the very headwaters where they were born, or sea turtles to the same beaches each year to lay their eggs?

Human beings depend on nature to meet their vital needs and are inevitably part of the complex network linking all biotic and abiotic elements of Earth's ecosystems. Yet, unlike the rest of living beings, our intelligence and social characteristics make our presence in ecosystems profoundly transformative, all too often disrupting the needs, habitats or ecosystems of many other species, and even undermining, whether inadvertently or deliberately, our own natural means of subsistence. As a telling example, we belong to a generation so detached from nature in certain respects that nocturnal light pollution allows only one third of humanity to see the Milky Way (Falchi *et al.*, 2016).

As knowledge advances regarding the influence of physical factors — such as those examined in this book: electromagnetic radiation pulses generated by lightning discharges during thunderstorms, as well as geomagnetic and solar activity — and their effects on human beings, nature reminds us once again of our true place: that of just another species, subject, like all others, to the vicissitudes of time. And in this case, we refer both to atmospheric time and to chronological time.

These electromagnetic waves (*sferics*) penetrate buildings with ease. It may therefore seem surprising that, isolated from nature as we appear to be by cement and brick, these natural influences —which feel so distant — can enter our bodies and brains without our realising it, altering our brainwaves and influencing, in one way or another, our physical state and our disposition to face the everyday challenges of life.

10.1 Evolutionary Advantages of Anticipating or Being Sensitive to Sferics

The Earth's magnetic field has also been essential for the evolution of life, as it provides a protective "shield" against harmful cosmic radiation and prevents our atmosphere from being eroded by the solar wind.
(Palmer *et al.*, 2003).

Over the course of life's history on Earth, rare events that episodically kill or reduce the fitness of a portion of individuals within a species can drive the evolution of mechanisms to avoid such mortality, through random mutations and natural selection. This is well known in the context of adaptation to disease. Living organisms can develop behaviours that enhance survival and fitness, such as the ability to escape predators or flee from fire. Many of these behaviours involve sophisticated pattern-recognition skills. Research over the past fifty years has shown that a large number of the complex behavioural responses exhibited by animals are under genetic control (Kirschvink, 2000).

It is likely that, throughout the evolution of animals and humans, there have been adaptive advantages associated with the ability to perceive in advance the signs that precede weather changes and earthquakes (*sferics*), which functioned as warning signals of certain risks or environmental alterations.

Animals seem to excel at the survival tasks that are vital to them; as such, they act as a kind of meteorological prophet, predicting the weather ahead of time — a quality already recognised by our ancestors (Baumer & Sönning, 2002). In traditional knowledge, observing animal behaviour has often helped predict weather conditions and, on occasion, earthquakes. Local elders, hunters, farmers and others whose livelihoods are deeply entwined with nature learn, through observation and experience, to notice particular signs reflected in the behaviour of animals within the natural environment of a given locality (Lakshmi *et al.*, 2014).

As seen in previous chapters, polarised *sferics* produced both by thunderstorms associated with cold fronts and by earthquakes can travel great distances, reflected between the ionosphere and the sea surface, especially at night. It is possible that, over the course of evolution, living beings adapted to detect them because of the advantage gained from knowing in advance the arrival of rain, bad weather or a catastrophe such as an earthquake.

This has been noted by other researchers, who have attributed the heightened bioactivity of low-frequency (ELF) pulses to the fact that living organisms were exposed, at the dawn of biological evolution on Earth, to intense thunderstorm activity and therefore to a high presence of *sferics* in the atmosphere (Panagopoulos & Balmori, 2017).

The "telecommunications" between all cells — and especially between the neurons of any living organism — are based precisely on these mechanisms of information transfer through highly specific signal tuning, present since the beginning of evolution (Baumer & Sönning, 2002). However, what may have become an adaptive advantage for early-warning detection during evolution has increasingly turned into an impediment in modern society.

People suffering from meteoropathy are affected by weather changes and may also become electrohypersensitive (EHS): they cannot tolerate artificial radiation and become extremely sensitive to natural sources as well, developing a sort of extreme allergy. Given the excellent suitability of *sferics* for remote detection or meteorological diagnosis, there exists the risk of overlap between natural and technological signals (from mobile telephony), and with it the real danger of synergistic effects, with medium- and long-term consequences for human, animal and plant health (Baumer & Sönning, 2002).

In Spain, as in other countries, telecommunications regulations have been drafted primarily in accordance with the interests of major corporations, facilitating the installation of antennas rather than safeguarding citizens' right to live in an environment free from electromagnetic pollution. Moreover, Spanish legislation does not require companies to hold civil liability insurance covering potential adverse health effects arising from such pollution. Ignoring warnings from the scientific community entails a serious risk: a society that refuses to listen to its experts inevitably moves towards disaster. The rollout of 5G technology, for instance, involves an unprecedented expansion in the number of potentially affected individuals, as it requires the installation of thousands of new antennas, many of them located very close to homes and workplaces

11
BY WAY OF A COROLLARY

Over the course of ten chapters, we have taken a descriptive journey through common observations of the effects of weather conditions and changes in the atmosphere on both animals and humans. We have examined the traditional explanations that science has attempted to offer for these curious or unusual observations, before presenting a more convincing account based on recent knowledge — drawing, among many other sources, on several scientific publications by the author.

Human beings, like other animals, are subject to the influence of meteorological phenomena. Feelings of dejection alternate with elevated mood and euphoria, as if driven by an invisible force. Certain anticipatory behaviours shown by animals in specific situations, before impending changes in the weather and even before particular natural disasters such as earthquakes, are well known, yet their biological basis remains unresolved. Equally striking are certain simultaneous events in human societies which, at first glance, may appear coincidental. The symptoms and pains of some chronic patients worsen with the arrival of cold, rain or changes in atmospheric pressure, and there are very significant individual differences in vulnerability to these factors.

Until quite recently, it was assumed that for animals to forecast forthcoming weather, they had to be within the air mass responsible for the atmospheric change and could therefore detect it only when it was already imminent and its characteristic conditions had begun to manifest. However, we now know that electrical discharges produced in a cold front with associated storms, even when located hundreds or thousands of kilometres away, generate electromagnetic impulses (*sferics*) that travel great distances at the speed of light, to which some people and animals are particularly sensitive.

This book examines current scientific findings to shed light on phenomena that remain largely unexplained. One of the chapters focuses on a symptom commonly associated with weather changes: headaches or migraines. Over five years, a detailed monitoring study was conducted with several individuals, relating the appearance of these episodes to the specific atmospheric conditions in which they occurred, using surface weather maps. The aim was to identify climatic patterns that may act as triggers and to explore possible explanations from a scientific perspective.

A review is also presented of the effects of technological electromagnetic radiation (which in some respects resembles natural radiation) on human beings, and the complex relationship between science and economics is analysed — a recurrent issue in environmental disciplines that often collide with powerful human interests. Evidence is shown of the effects of electromagnetic radiation on animals and plants, and of how living organisms can serve as natural sensors of environmental degradation.

The ability of animals to predict seismic movements is then described, along with the electromagnetic agents involved in this perceptive capacity, which turn out to be similar to *sferics* of atmospheric origin. Peaks in variations of electromagnetic signals are detected a few days before an earthquake and persist for several days afterwards. Such polarised pulses are perceived by a wide range of species, as well as by sensitive individuals, which may perfectly explain the early warnings shown by many different groups of animals reported in the scientific literature. A detailed explanation is provided of how *sferics* modify the flow of ions into and out of cells through membrane channels.

The growing number of papers published in recent years reveals the significant influence of geophysical factors — changes in solar activity and geomagnetic disturbances — on physiological, biological and health parameters in healthy individuals. It has been shown that marked variations in these parameters can cause health problems in living organisms, and that a proportion of the population, estimated at between 10% and 15%, is predisposed to adverse health effects caused by geomagnetic fluctuations. There are also non-coincidental similarities between electrosensitivity and meteoropathy, both of which affect a substantial percentage of people.

Polarised *sferics* produced by thunderstorms associated with cold fronts, as well as by earthquakes, can travel great distances, reflected between the ionosphere and the sea surface, especially at night. In a stable geomagnetic environment, low-frequency electromagnetic pulses originate from the atmosphere (*sferics*) and are governed mainly by meteorological factors (especially cold fronts). However, when solar storms or other factors alter the geomagnetic characteristics of the Earth — for example, earthquakes or solar and cosmic radiation — the effects of radiation from different sources overlap, affecting living organisms.

It is likely that organisms have adapted to detect these signals in the course of evolution, because of the advantage that early knowledge of incoming rain and bad weather — or the anticipation of serious catastrophes such as earthquakes — may provide.

BIBLIOGRAPHY

Abdel-Rassoul, G.; El-Fateh, O. A.; Salem, M. A.; Michael, A.; Farahat, F.; El-Batanouny, M., y Salem, E. (2007). «Neurobehavioral effects among inhabitants around mobile phone base stations». *Neurotoxicology*, 28(2), 434-440.

Adams, J. A.; Galloway, T. S.; Mondal, D.; Esteves, S. C., y Mathews, F. (2014). «Effect of mobile telephones on sperm quality: a systematic review and meta-analysis». *Environment international*, 70, 106-112.

Adelaja, O. J.; Ande, A. T.; Abdulraheem, G. D.; Oluwakorode, I. A.; Oladipo, O. A., y Oluwajobi, A. O. (2021). «Distribution, diversity and abundance of some insects around a telecommunication mast in Ilorin, Kwara State, Nigeria». *Bulletin of the National Research Centre*, 45, 1-7.

Alberts, B.; Bray, D.; Lewis, J.; Raff, M.; Roberts, K., y Watson, J. D. (1994). *Molecular Biology of the Cell*. Garlang Publishing: New York.

Alvarado-Rybak, M.; Toro, F.; Escobar-Dodero, J.; Kinsley, A. C.; Sepúlveda, M. A.; Capella, J., y Mardones, F. O. «50 Years of Cetacean Strandings Reveal a Concerning Rise in Chilean Patagonia». *Sci. Rep.* 2020, 10, 9511.55

Asada, T.; Baba, H.; Kawazoe, M., y Sugiura, M. (2001). «An attempt to delineate very low frequency electromagnetic signals associated with earthquakes». *Earth, planets and space*, 53(1), 55-62.

Auliciems, A. y DiBartolo, L. (1995). «Domestic violence in a subtropical environment: Police calls and weather in Brisbane». *International Journal of Biometeorology*, 39(1), 34-39.

Babayev, E. S. y Allahverdiyeva, A. A. (2007). «Effects of geomagnetic activity variations on the physiological and psychological state of functionally healthy humans: some results of Azerbaijani studies». *Advances in Space Research*, 40(12), 1941-1951.

Balmori, A. (2004). «¿Pueden afectar las microondas pulsadas emitidas por las antenas de telefonía a los árboles y otros vegetales?». *Ecosistemas*, 13(3). Disponible en https://www.revistaecosistemas.net/index.php/ecosistemas/article/view/534.

— (2005). «Possible effects of electromagnetic fields from phone masts on a population of white stork (*Ciconia ciconia*)». *Electromagnetic Biology and Medicine*, 24(2), 109-119.

— y Hallberg, Ö. (2007). «The urban decline of the house sparrow (*Passer domesticus*): a possible link with electromagnetic radiation». *Electromagnetic Biology and Medicine*, 26(2), 141-151.

— (2009). «Electromagnetic pollution from phone masts. Effects on wildlife». *Pathophysiology*, 16(2-3), 191-199.

— (2010). «Mobile phone mast effects on common frog (*Rana temporaria*) tadpoles: the city turned into a laboratory». *Electromagnetic Biology and Medicine*, 29(1-12), 31-35.

— (2014). «Electrosmog and species conservation». *Science of the Total Environment*, 496, 314-316.

— (2015). «Anthropogenic radiofrequency electromagnetic fields as an emerging threat to wildlife orientation». *Science of the Total Environment*, 518, 58-60.

— (2017). «Advances on the group composition, mating system, roosting and flight behaviour of the European free-tailed bat (*Tadarida teniotis*)». *Mammalia*.

— (2021). «Electromagnetic radiation as an emerging driver factor for the decline of insects». *Sci. Total. Environ.*, 767, 144913.

— y Balmori-de la Puente, A. (2024). «Potential Effects of Anthropogenic Radiofrequency Radiation on Cetaceans». *Radiation*, 4(1), 1-16. Disponible en https://doi.org/10.3390/radiation4010001.

Balsamo, V.; Sirtori, P. G.; Miani, J. A.; Di, A. F.; Franceschini, R.; Mauro, F., y Grassi, G. (1992). «Meteoropathy: a syndrome continuously on the increase». *La Clínica Terapéutica*, 141(7), 3-8.

Bandara, P. y Carpenter, D. O. (2018). «Planetary electromagnetic pollution: it is time to assess its impact». *The Lancet Planetary Health*, 2(12), e512-e514.

Batellier, F.; Couty, I.; Picard, D., y Brillard, J. P. (2008). «Effects of exposing chicken eggs to a cell phone in "call" position over the entire incubation period». *Theriogenology*, 69(6), 737-745.

Baumer H. y Sönning, W. (2002). *Das natürliche ImpulsFrequenzspektrum der Atmosphäre (CD-Sferics a.t.B.) und seine biologische Wirksamkeit.*

Becker, W. J. (2010). «Weather and migraine: can so many patients be wrong?». *Cephalalgia*, 31 (4), 387-390.

Belpomme, D. y Irigaray, P. (2022). «Why Electrohypersensitivity and Related Symptoms Are Caused by Non-ionizing Man-Made Electromagnetic Fields: an Overview and Medical Assessment». *Environmental Research*, 113374.

Bernatzky, A. (1986). «Elektromagnetischer Smog. Feind des Lebens». *Der Naturarzt*, 11, 22-25.

Berk, M.; Dodd, S., y Henry, M. (2006). «Do ambient electromagnetic fields affect behaviour? A demonstration of the relationship between geomagnetic storm activity and suicide». *Bioelectromagnetics*, 27(2), 151-155.

Bhargava, N.; Katiyar, V. K.; Sharma, M. L., y Pradhan, P. (2009). «Earthquake prediction through animal behavior: A review». *Indian Journal of Biomechanics*, 7, 8.

Bhat, T. A. y Singh, D. (2019). «Effect of mobile tower radiation on avian fauna: A case study of Lolab Valley, Kupwara Jammu and Kashmir». *JETIR*, 6, 570-576.

Bhattacharya, R. y Roy, R. (2013). «Impacts of Communication Towers on Avians: A Review». *IJECT*, 4, 137-139.

Bose, S.; Roy, R.; Chakraborti, U.; Samanta, R.; Jana, S.; Mondal, T., y Bhattacharya, S. C. R. (2020). «Impressions of high frequency radio-waves from cell phone towers on birds: A base-line study». *J. Multidiscip. Res.*, 1, 54-62.

Brezowsky, H. (1965). «Über die Beeinflussung der Samenkeimung durch atmosphärische Vorgänge. Archiv für meteorologie». *Geophysik und Bioklimatologie*, Serie B, 13(4), 521-530.

Burch, J. B.; Reif, J. S., y Yost, M. G. (1999). «Geomagnetic disturbances are associated with reduced nocturnal excretion of a melatonin metabolite in humans». *Neuroscience letters*, 266(3), 209-212.

Butke, P. y Sheridan, S. C. (2010). «An analysis of the relationship between weather and aggressive crime in Cleveland, Ohio». *Weather, Climate, and Society*, 2(2), 127-139.

Cammaerts, M. C.; De Doncker, P.; Patris, X.; Bellens, F.; Rachidi, Z., y Cammaerts, D. (2012). «GSM 900 MHz radiation inhibits ants' association between food sites and encountered cues». *Electromagnetic biology and medicine*, 31(2), 151-165.

Cherry, N. (2002). «Schumann Resonances, a plausible biophysical mechanism for the human health effects of Solar/Geomagnetic Activity». *Natural Hazards*, 26(3), 279-331.

— (2002). *Actual or potential effects of ELF and RF/MW radiation on enhancing violence and homicide, and accelerating aging of human, animal or plant cells.* Human Sciences Department. Lincoln University Canterbury: New Zealand. Disponible en http://researcharchive.lincoln.ac.nz/handle/10182/4006.

Chu, M. K.; Song, H. G.; Kim, C., y Lee, B. C. (2011). «Clinical features of headache associated with mobile phone use: a cross-sectional study in university students». *BMC neurology*, 11(1), 115.

Coombs, E. J.; Deaville, R.; Sabin, R. C.; Allan, L.; O'Connell, M.; Berrow, S., y Cooper, N. (2019). «What can cetacean stranding records tell us? A study of UK and Irish cetacean diversity over the past 100 years». *Mar. Mammal Sci.*, 35, 1527-1555.

Coughran, D. K.; Gales, N. J., y Smith, H. C. (2013). «A note on the spike in recorded mortality of humpback whales (*Megaptera novaeangliae*) in Western Australia». *J. Cetacean Res. Manag.*, 13, 105-108.53.

Cucurachi, S.; Tamis, W. L. M.; Vijver, M. G.; Peijnenburg, W. J. G. M.; Bolte, J. F. B., y De Snoo, G. R. (2013). «A review of the ecological effects of radiofrequency electromagnetic fields (RF-EMF)». *Environment International*, 51, 116-140.

Da Luigi Janiri, S.; Spinetti, G.; Mazza, M., y Di Nicola, M. (2013). «Meteoropathy: a new disease». *Archivio*, 1(1-2). Disponible en http://www.psicocardio.org/index.php?option=com_content&view=article&id=28:meteoropathy-a-new-disease&catid=38:psychiatry-and-quality-of-life&Itemid=132.

Dadam, D.; Robinson, R. A.; Clements, A.; Peach,W. J.; Bennett, M.; Rowcliffe, J. M., y Cunningham, A. A. (2019). «Avian malaria-mediated population decline of a widespread iconic bird species». *R. Soc. Open Sci.*, 6, 182197.

Davoudi, M.; Brössner, C., y Kuber, W. (2002). «Der Einfluss elektromagnetischer wellen auf die Spermienmotilität». *Journal für Urologie und Urogynäkologie*, 9, 18-22.

De, S. S.; De, B. K.; Bandyopadhyay, B.; Paul, S.; De, D.; Barui, S., y Das, T. K. (2011). «Studies on the precursors of an earthquake as the vlf electromagnetic sferics». *Rome J. Phys*, 56 (9-10), 1208-1227.

Dimitrova, S.; Mustafa, F. R.; Stoilova, I.; Babayev, E. S., y Kazimov, E. A. (2009). «Possible influence of solar extreme events and related geomagnetic disturbances on human cardio-vascular state: Results of collaborative Bulgarian-Azerbaijani studies». *Advances in space research*, 43(4), 641-648.

Dologlou, E. (2010). «Recent aspects on possible interrelation between precursory electric signals and anomalous bioeffects». *Natural Hazards and Earth System Sciences*, 10(9), 1951-1955.

Dovrat, A.; Berenson, R.; Bormusov, E.; Lahav, A.; Lustman, T.; Sharon, N., y L. Schachter (2005). «Localized Effects of Microwave Radiation on the Intact Eye Lens in Culture Conditions». *Bioelectromagnetics*, 26, 398-405.

Eger, H.; Hagen, K.; Lucas, B.; Vogel, P., y Voit, H. (2004). «Einfluss der räumlichen Nähe von Mobilfunksendeanlagen auf die Krebsinzidenz». *Unwelt medizin gesellschaft*, 17, 326-332.

— y Jahn, M. (2010). «Spezifische Symptome und Mobilfunkstrahlung in Selbitz (Bayern) Evidenz für eine Dosiswirkungsbeziehung». *Umwelt Medizin Gesellschaft*, 2, 130-9.

Egilman, D. S. y Bohme, R. (2005). «Over a barrel: corporate corruption of science and its effects on workers and the environment». *International Journal of Occupational and Environmental Health*, 11(4), 331-337.

Engels, S.; Schneider, N. L.; Lefeldt, N.; Hein, C. M.; Zapka, M.; Michalik, A.; Elbers, D.; Kittel, A.; Hore, P. J., y Mouritsen, H. (2014). «Anthropogenic electromagnetic noise disrupts magnetic compass orientation in a migratory bird». *Nature*, 509, 353-356.

Everaert, J. y Bauwens, D. (2007). «A possible effect of electromagnetic radiation from mobile phone base stations on the number of breeding house sparrows (*Passer domesticus*)». *Electromagnetic biology and medicine*, 26(1), 63-72.

Falcioni, L.; Bua, L.; Tibaldi, E.; Lauriola, M.; De Angelis, L.; Gnudi, F., y Belpoggi, F. (2018). «Report of final results regarding brain and heart tumors in Sprague-Dawley rats exposed from prenatal life until natural death to mobile phone radiofrequency field representative of a 1.8 GHz GSM base station environmental emission». *Environ. Res.* 165, 496-503.

Falchi, F, P.; Cinzano, D.; Duriscoe, C. C. M.; Kyba, C. D.; Elvidge, K.; Baugh, B. A.; Portnov, N. A.; Rybnikova, y Furgoni, R. (2016). «The new world atlas of artificial night sky brightness». *Science Advances*, 1-26.

Ferasyi, T. R.; Sabri, M.; Hamdani, H.; Azhari, A.; Amiruddin, A.; Erwin, E., y Faber, R. (2013). «An indication of african catfish's (*Clarias gariepinus*) behavioral changes as a response for increased seismic activity». *Journal Natural*, 13(1).

Ferrari, T. E. (2014). «Magnets, magnetic field fluctuations and geomagnetic disturbances impair the homing ability of honey bee (*Apis m.*)». *J. Apicult Res.* IBRA 53, 452-456.

Foster, K. R. y Finch, E. D. (1974). «Microwave hearing: Evidence for thermoacoustic auditory stimulation by pulsed microwaves». *Science*, 185, 256-258.

Frey, A. H. (1998). «Headaches from cellular telephones: are they real and what are the impacts». *Environ Health Perspect*, 106, 101-103.

Galeev, A. L. (2000). «The effects of microwave radiation from mobile telephones on humans and animals». *Neurosci. Behav. Physiol.*, 30, 187-194.

García Callejo, F. J.; García Callejo, F.; Peña Santamaría, J.; Alonso Castañeira, I.; Sebastián Gil, E., y Marco Algarra, J. (2005). «Nivel auditivo y uso intensivo de teléfonos móviles». *Acta Otorrinolaringol. Esp.*, 56, 187-191.

Golomb, B. A. (2018). «Diplomats' mystery illness and pulsed radiofrequency/microwave radiation». *Neural Comput.*, 30 (11), 2882-2985.

Gómez-Perretta, C.; Navarro, E. A.; Segura, J., y Portolés, M. (2013). «Subjective symptoms related to GSM radiation from mobile phone base stations: a cross-sectional study». *BMJ open*, 3(12), e003836.

Gordon, C. y Berk, M. (2003). «The effect of geomagnetic storms on suicide». *African Journal of Psychiatry*, 6(3).

Granger, J.; Walkowicz, L.; Fitak, R., y Johnsen, S. (2020). «Gray whales strand more often on days with increased levels of atmospheric radio-frequency noise». *Current Biology*, 30(4), R155-R156.

Granlund-Lind, R. y Lind, J. (2004). *Black on white. Voices and witnesses about electro-hypersensitivity. The swedish experience*. Mimers Brunn: Sweden.

Grant, R. A. y Halliday, T. (2010). «Predicting the unpredictable; evidence of pre-seismic anticipatory behaviour in the common toad». *Journal of Zoology*, 281(4), 263-271.

—; Halliday, T.; Balderer, W. P.; Leuenberger, F.; Newcomer, M.; Cyr, G., y Freund, F. T. (2011). «Ground water chemistry changes before major earthquakes and possible effects on animals». *International Journal of Environmental Research and Public Health*, 8(6), 1936-1956.

—; Raulin, J. P., y Freund, F. T. (2015). «Changes in animal activity prior to a major (M= 7) earthquake in the Peruvian Andes». *Physics and Chemistry of the Earth, Parts A/B/C*, 85, 69-77.

Hallberg, O. y Johansson, O. (2004). «Malignant melanoma of the skin. Not a sunshine story!». *Med Sci Monit*, 10, 336-340.

— y Oberfeld, G. (2006). «Letter to the editor: will we all become electrosensitive?». *Electromagnetic Biology and Medicine*, 25(3), 189-191.

Hansen, C.; Lundh, A.; Rasmussen, K.; Gøtzsche, P. C., y Hróbjartsson, A. (2017). «The influence of industry funding and other financial conflicts of interest on the outcomes and quality of systematic reviews». *Peer Review Congress*.

Harremoes, P.; Gee, D.; MacGarvin, M.; Stirling, A.; Keys, J.; Wynne, B., y Vaz, S. G. (eds.) (2013). *The Precautionary Principle in the 20th Century: Late Lessons from Early Warnings*. Routledge: London.

Hardell, L.; Hallquist, A.; Hansson, K.; Carlberg, M.; Pahlson, A., y Lilja. A. (2002). «Cellular and cordless telephones and the risk for brain tumours». *European Journal of Cancer Prevention*, 11, 377-386.

Hässig, M.; Wullschleger, M.; Naegeli, H.; Kupper, J.; Spiess, B.; Kuster, N., y Murbach, M. (2014). «Influence of non ionizing radiation of base stations on the activity of redox proteins in bovines». *BMC Veterinary Research*, 10(1), 136.

Höppe, P. (1997). «Aspects of human biometerology in past, present and future». *International Journal of Biometeorology*, 40(1), 19-23.

Hsu, C. Y.; Ko, F. Y.; Li, C. W.; Fann, K., y Lue, J. T. (2007). «Magnetoreception system in honeybees (*Apis mellifera*)». *PloS one*, 2(4), e395.

Hwang, H. S.; Lee, H.; Yoon, S. Y.; Kim, J. S.; Jeong, K.; Kronbichler, A.; y Yon, D. K. (2025). «Global burden of vaccine-associated kidney injury using an international pharmacovigilance database». *Scientific Reports*, 15(1), 5177.

Hutchison, Z. L.; Gill, A. B.; Sigray, P.; He, H., y King, J. W. (2020). «Anthropogenic electromagnetic fields (EMF) influence the behaviour of bottom-dwelling marine species». *Sci. Rep.*, 10, 4219.

Hutter, H. P.; Moshammer, H., y Kundi, M. (2002). «Mobile telephone base-stations: efects on health and wellbeing». *2nd International workshop on biological effects of EMFs*, Rhodes (Greece), 1, 344-352.

Huss, A.; Egger, M.; Hug, K.; Huwiler-Müntener, K., y Röösli, M. (2006). «Source of funding and results of studies of health effects of mobile phone use: systematic review of experimental studies». *Environmental Health Perspectives*, 115(1), 1-4.

Hyland, G. J. (2000). «Physics and biology of mobile telephony». *The Lancet*, 356(9244), 1833-1836.

— (2001). «Los efectos fisiológicos y medioambientales de la radiación electromagnética no ionizante». *Resumen de opciones y Síntesis. PE*, (297.574).

Ikeya, M.; Yamanaka, C.; Mattsuda, T.; Sasaoka, H.; Ochiai, H.; Huang, Q., y Nakagawa, T. (2000). «Electromagnetic pulses generated by compression of granitic rocks and animal behavior». *Episodes*, 23(4), 262-265.

Jacobi, E. (1977). «Untersuchungen zur Pathophysiologie der Thrombozytenadhäsivität. Habilitationsschrift». *Med. Fak.* Universität Düsseldorf.

Jeffery, G.; Fosbury, R.; Barrett, E.; Hogg, C.; Carmona, M. R., y Powner, M. B. (2025). «Longer wavelengths in sunlight pass through the human body and have a systemic impact which improves vision». *Scientific Reports*, 15(1), 24435.

Johnson Liakouris, A. G. (1998). «Radiofrequency (RF) Sickness in the Lilienfeld Study: an effect of modulated microwaves?». *Archives of Environmental Health: An International Journal*, 53(3), 236-238.

Khabarova, O. V. y Dimitrova, S. (2008). «Some proves of integrated influence of geomagnetic activity and weather changes on human health». *ArXiv preprint arXiv:0810.0457.*

Khurana, V. G.; Hardell, L.; Everaert, J.; Bortkiewicz, A.; Carlberg, M., y Ahonen, M. (2010). «Epidemiological evidence for a health risk from mobile phone base stations». *International journal of occupational and environmental health*, 16(3), 263-267.

Kirschvink, J. L. (2000). «Earthquake prediction by animals: Evolution and sensory perception». *Bulletin of the Seismological Society of America*, 90(2), 312-323.

Koizumi, T., y Ono, M. (2025). «Cardiac Multiple Micro-Scars: An Autopsy Study». *Case Reports*, 30(5), 103083.

Kolodynski, A. A. y Kolodynska, V. V. (1996). «Motor and psychological functions of school children living in the area of the Skrunda Radio Location Station in Latvia». *Sci. Total Environ.*, 180 (1), 87-93.

Kramarenko, A. V. y Tan, U. (2003). «Effects of high frequency electromagnetic fields on human EEG: a brain mapping study». *Int. J. Neurosci.* 113, 1007-1019.

Kveton, V. (1991). «Weather fronts and acute myocardial infarction». *International Journal of Biometeorology*, 35(1), 10-17.

Lai, H. y Singh, N. P. (1995). «Acute low-intensity microwave exposure increases DNA single-strand breaks in rat brain cells». *Bioelectromagnetics*, 16, 207-210.

Lakshmi, K. R.; Nagesh, Y., y Krishna, M. V. (2014). «Analysis on Predicting Earthquakes through an Abnormal Behavior of Animals». *International Journal of Scientific & Engineering Research*, 5(4), 845-857.

Lawrence, A.; Rawls, M. L.; Jah, M.; Boley, A.; Di Vruno, F.; Garrington, S., y McCaughrean, M. (2022). «The case for space environmentalism». *Nature Astronomy*, 6(4), 428-435.

Lázaro, A.; Chroni, A.; Tscheulin, T.; Devalez, J.; Matsoukas, C., y Petanidou, T. (2016). «Electromagnetic radiation ofmobile telecommunication antennas affects the abundance and composition of wild pollinators». *J. Insect Conserv.*, 20, 315-324.

Le Beau, J. L. y Corcoran, W. T. (1990). «Changes in calls for police service with changes in routine activities and the arrival and passage of weather fronts». *Journal of Quantitative Criminology*, 6(3), 269-291.

Leal Hernández, M.; Abellán Alemán, J., y Casas Pina, M. (2005). «Telefonía móvil. ¿Una apuesta con nuestra salud?». *Atención Primaria*, 35(8), 415-8.

Leszczynski, D.; Joenväärä, S.; Reivinen, J., y Kuokka, R. (2002). «Non-thermal activation of the hsp27/p38MAPK stress pathway by mobile phone radiation in human endothelial cells: Molecular mechanism for cancer- and blood-brain barrier-related effects». *Differentiation*, 70, 120-129.

Levitt, B. B. y Lai, H. (2010). «Biological effects from exposure to electromagnetic radiation emitted by cell tower base stations and other antenna arrays». *Environmental Reviews*, 18(NA), 369-395.

—; Lai, H. C., y Manville, A. M. (2022). «Effects of non-ionizing electromagnetic fields on flora and fauna, part 1. Rising ambient EMF levels in the environment». *Rev. Environ. Health*, 37, 81-122.

—; Lai, H. C., y Manville, A. M. (2022). «Effects of non-ionizing electromagnetic fields on flora and fauna, Part 2 impacts: How species interact with natural and man-made EMF». *Rev. Environ. Health*, 37, 327-406.

Li, Y.; Liu, Y.; Jiang, Z.; Guan, J.; Yi, G.; Cheng, S., y Wang, Z. (2009). «Behavioral change related to Wenchuan devastating earthquake in mi ce». *Bioelectromagnetics*, 30(8), 613-620.

Lilienfeld, A. M.; Tonascia, J.; Tonascia, S., *et al.* (1978). *Foreign Service Health Status Study*. Department of State, Washington, D. C. Final report contract no. 6025-619037 (NTS publication PB-288163).

Lin, J. C. (2019). «The significance of primary tumors in the NTP study of chronic rat exposure to cell phone radiation [health matters]». *IEEE Microwave Magazine*, 20(11), 18-21.

Lonn, S.; Ahlbom, A.; Hall, P., y Feychting, M. (2004). «Mobile Phone Use and the Risk of Acoustic Neuroma». *Epidemiology*, 15(6), 653-659.

López, A.; Santos, M. B.; Pierce, G. J.; González, A. F.; Valeiras, X., y Guerra, A. (2002). «Trends in strandings and by-catch of marine mammals in north-west Spain during the 1990s. J». *Mar. Biol. Assoc.*, 82, 513-521.58

Lousada Arochena, J. F. y Ron Latas, R. P. (2024). «Sensibilidad química múltiple y electrohipersensibilidad: tratamiento jurídico laboral y perspectiva de género». *Revista de Derecho de la Seguridad Social*, Laborum, (39), 35-50.

Lundh, A.; Lexchin, J.; Mintzes, B.; Schroll, J. B., y Bero, L. (2017). «Industry sponsorship and research outcome». *Cochrane Database of Systematic Reviews*, Issue 2. Art. n.º MR000033.

Mackensen, S. V.; Hoeppe, P.; Maarouf, A.; Tourigny, P., y Nowak, D. (2005). «Prevalence of weather sensitivity in Germany and Canada». *International journal of biometeorology*, 49(3), 156-166.

Malin, S. R. C. y Srivastava, B. J. (1979). «Correlation between heart attacks and magnetic activity». *Nature*, 277(5698), 646.

Martin, G. V.; Houle, T.; Nicholson, R.; Peterlin, A., y Martin, V. T. (2013). «Lightning and its association with the frequency of headache in migraineurs: An observational cohort study». *Cephalalgia*, 33(6), 375-383.

Martínez-Carpio, P. A. (2003). «Biometeorología y bioclimatología clínica: fundamentos, aplicaciones clínicas y estado actual de estas ciencias». *Atención Primaria*, 32(5), 300-305.

Mazza, M.; Di Nicola, M.; Catalano, V.; Callea, A.; Martinotti, G.; Harnic, D., y Janiri, L. (2012). «Description and validation of a questionnaire for the detection of meteoropathy and meteorosensitivity: the METEO-Q». *Comprehensive psychiatry*, 53(1), 103-106.

Mendoza, B. y De la Peña, S. S. (2010). «Solar activity and human health at middle and low geomagnetic latitudes in Central America». *Advances in space research*, 46(4), 449-459.

Migdał, P.; Plotnik, M.; Bie'nkowski, P.; Berbe'c, E.; Latarowski, K.; Białecka, N., y Murawska, A. (2025). «The Influence of an Electromagnetic Field at a Radiofrequency of 900 MHz on the Behavior of a Honey Bee». *Agriculture*, 15, 1266. Disponible en https://doi.org/10.3390/agriculture15121266.

Mohring, B.; Henry, P. Y.; Jiguet, F.; Malher, F., y Angelier, F. (2021). «Investigating temporal and spatial correlates of the sharp decline of an urban exploiter bird in a large European city». *Urban Ecosyst.*, 24, 501-513.

Molina-Montenegro, M. A.; Acuña-Rodríguez, I. S.; Ballesteros, G. I.; Baldelomar, M.; Torres-Díaz, C.; Broitman, B. R.; y Vázquez, D. P. (2023). «Electromagnetic fields disrupt the pollination service by honeybees». *Science Advances*, 9(19), eadh1455.

Møller, A. P. (2019). «Parallel declines in abundance of insects and insectivorous birds in Denmark over 22 years». *Ecology and Evolution*, 9, 6581-6587.

Murgui, E. y Macias, A. (2010). «Changes in the House Sparrow Passer domesticus population in Valencia (Spain) from 1998 to 2008». *Bird Study*, 57, 281-288.

Nagao, T.; Enomoto, Y.; Fujinawa, Y.; Hata, M.; Hayakawa, M.; Huang, Q., y Uyeda, S. (2002). «Electromagnetic anomalies associated with 1995 Kobe earthquake». *Journal of Geodynamics*, 33(4-5), 401-411.

National Academies of Sciences (2020). *Engineering, and medicine. An assessment of illness in US government employees and their families at overseas embassies.* Disponible en https://doi.org/10.17226/25889.

Navarro, E. A.; Segura, J.; Portolés, M., y Gómez Perretta, C. (2003). «The microwave Syndrome: A preliminary Study in Spain». *Electromagnetic Biology and Medicine*, 22, 161-169.

Nicholls, B. y Racey, P. A. (2009). «The aversive effect of electromagnetic radiation on foraging bats. A possible means of discouraging bats from approaching wind turbines». *PLoS One*, 4(7), e6246.

Oberfeld, G.; Navarro, E.; Portoles, M.; Maestu C., y Gómez-Perretta, C. (2004). «The Microwave Syndrome. Further Aspects of a Spanish Study». *EBEA Congres Kos-Greece.*

Odemer, R. y Odemer, F. (2018). «Effects of radiofrequency electromagnetic radiation (RF-EMF) on honey bee queen development and mating success». *Science of the Total Environment*, 661, 553-562.

Pall, M. L. (2013). «Electromagnetic fields act via activation of voltage-gated calcium channels to produce beneficial or adverse effects». *Journal of Cellular and Molecular Medicine*, 17(8), 958-965.

Palmer, S. J.; Rycroft, M. J., y Cermack, M. (2006). «Solar and geomagnetic activity, extremely low frequency magnetic and electric fields and human health at the Earth's surface». *Surveys in Geophysics*, 27(5), 557-595.

Panagopoulos, D. J.; Messini, N.; Karabarbounis, A.; Philippetis, A. L., y Margaritis, L. H. (2000). «A mechanism for action of oscillating electric fields on cells». *Biochemical and biophysical research communications*, 272(3), 634-640.

—; Karabarbounis, A., y Margaritis, L. H. (2004). «Effect of GSM 900 MHz mobile phone radiation on the reproductive capacity of Drosophila melanogaster». *Electromagnetic Biology and Medicine*, 23, 29-43.

—; Johansson, O., y Carlo, G. L. (2015). «Polarization: a key difference between man-made and natural electromagnetic fields, in regard to biological activity». *Scientific reports*, 5, 14914.

— y Balmori, A. (2017). «On the biophysical mechanism of sensing atmospheric discharges by living organisms». *Science of The Total Environment*, 599, 2026-2034.

—; Balmori, A., y Chrousos, G. P. (2020). «On the biophysical mechanism of sensing upcoming earthquakes by animals». *Science of the Total Environment*, 717, 136989.

—; Karabarbounis, A., y Chrousos, G. P. (2024). «Biophysical mechanism of animal magnetoreception, orientation and navigation». *Scientific Reports*, 14(1), 1-16.

—; Yakymenko, I.; De Iuliis, G. N., y Chrousos, G. P. (2025). «A Comprehensive Mechanism of Biological and Health Effects of Anthropogenic Extremely Low Frequency and Wireless Communication Electromagnetic Fields». *Frontiers in Public Health*, 13, 1585441.

Papailiou, M.; Mavromichalaki, H.; Kudela, K.; Stetiarova, J., y Dimitrova, S. (2011). «Effect of geomagnetic disturbances on physiological parameters: an investigation on aviators». *Advances in Space Research*, 48(9), 1545-1550.

Paracelso (1529, ed. 2014). *Das Buch Paragranum*. Henricus: Berlin.

Patone, M.; Mei, X. W.; Handunnetthi, L.; Dixon, S.; Zaccardi, F.; Shankar-Hari, M.; y Hippisley-Cox, J. (2022). «Risks of myocarditis, pericarditis, and cardiac arrhythmias associated with COVID-19 vaccination or SARS-CoV-2 infection». *Nature Medicine*, 28(2), 410-422.

Persinger, M. A. (1974). «ELF electric and magnetic field effects: The patterns and the problems», en *ELF and VLF electromagnetic field effects* (pp. 275-310). Springer: Boston, Massachusetts.

— (1980). *The weather matrix and human behavior*. Praeger Publishers: Westport, Connecticut.

Pessi, A. T. y Businger, S. (2009). «Relationships among lightning, precipitation, and hydrometeor characteristics over the North Pacific Ocean». *Journal of Applied Meteorology and Climatology*, 48(4), 833-848.

—; Businger, S.; Cummins, K. L.; Demetriades, N. W. S.; Murphy, M., y Pifer, B. (2009). «Development of a long-range lightning detection network for the Pacific: Construction, calibration, and performance». *Journal of Atmospheric and Oceanic Technology*, 26(2), 145-166.

Phillips, J. y Painter, M. (2022). «Small differences in weak electromagnetic fields disrupt magnetic compass orientation of C57 BL/6 mice (*Rodentia: Muridae*)». *Lynx new series*, 53, 219-234.

Plank, Max (1947). *Scientific Autobiography and Other Papers*, Greenwood Pub. Group: New York.

Reiter, R. (1960). *Meteorobiologie und Elektrizität der Atmosphäre*. Akademische Verlagsges Geest & Portig: Leipzig.

Sainudeen Sahib, S. (2011). «Impact of mobile phone on the density of honey bees». *Munis Entomology & Zoology*, 6 (1), 396-399.

Sakraoui, D.; Ziane, N.; Ghalem, R.; Boukheroufa, M., y Habbachi, W. (2023). «Is there an effect of electromagnetic waves from base stations on the breeding success of Ciconia ciconia ciconia in Algeria?». *Biosystems Diversity*, 31(4), 493-499.

Salford, L. G.; Brun, A. E.; Eberhardt, J. L.; Malmgren, L., y Persson, B. R. (2003). «Nerve cell damage in mammalian brain after exposure to microwaves from GSM mobile phones». *Environmental Health Perspectives*, 111(7), 881.

Sánchez-Bayo, F. y Wyckhuys, K. A. (2019). «Worldwide decline of the entomofauna: a review of its drivers». *Biol. Conserv.*, 232, 8-27.

Santini, R.; Santini, P.; Le Ruz, P.; Danze, J. M., y Seigne, M. (2003). «Survey Study of People Living in the Vicinity of Cellular Phone Base Stations». *Electromagnetic Biology and Medicine*, 22, 41-49.

Schaal, R. B. (1988). «An evaluation of the animal-behavior theory for earthquake prediction». *California Geology*, 41(2), 41-45.

Schienle, A.; Stark, R., y Vaitl, D. (2001). «Sferics provoke changes in EEG power». *International journal of neuroscience*, 107(1-2), 87-102.

— (2006). «Biological Effects of Very Low Frequency (VLF) Atmospherics in Humans: A Review». *Journal of Scientific Explorations*, 12 (3), 6.

Shahbazi-Gahrouei, D.; Karbalae, M.; Moradi, H. A., y Baradaran-Ghahfarokhi, M. (2014). «Health effects of living near mobile phone base transceiver station (BTS) antennae: a report from Isfahan, Iran». *Electromagnetic biology and medicine*, 33(3), 206-210.

Sheldrake, R. (2005). «Listen to the Animals». *The Ecologist*, 35(2), 18-20.

Shende, V. A. y Patil, K. G. (2015). «Electromagnetic radiations: A possible impact on population of house sparrow (*Passer Domesticus*)». *Eng. Int.*, 3, 45-52.

Singh, R.; Kour, D. N.; Ahmad, F.; Sahi, D. N. (2013). «The causes of decline of House Sparrow (Passer domesticus, Linnaeus 1758) in urban and suburban areas of Jammu Region J&K». *Mun. Ent. Zool.*, 8, 803-811.

Smith-Roe, S. L.; Wyde, M. E.; Stout, M. D.; Winters, J. W.; Hobbs, C. A.; Shepard, K. G., y Witt, K. L. (2020). «Evaluation of the genotoxicity of cell phone radiofrequency radiation in male and female rats and mice following subchronic exposure». *Environ. Mol. Mutagen.*, 61 (2), 276-290.

Sonzogni, L.; Al-Choboq, J.; Combemale, P.; Massardier-Pilonchéry, A.; Bouchet, A.; May, P.; Doré, J. F.; Debouzy, J. C.; Bourguignon, M.; Dréan, Y. L., *et al.* (2025). «Skin Fibroblasts from Individuals Self-Diagnosed as Electrosensitive Reveal Two Distinct Subsets with Delayed Nucleoshuttling of the ATM Protein in Common». *Int. J. Mol. Sci.*, 26, 4792. Disponible en https://doi.org/10.3390/ijms26104792.

Starkey, S. J. (2016). «Inaccurate official assessment of radiofrequency safety by the Advisory Group on Non-ionising Radiation». *Reviews on Environmental Health*, 31(4), 493-503.

Stoilova, I. y Dimitrova, S. (2008). «Geophysical variables and human health and behavior». *Journal of Atmospheric and Solar-Terrestrial Physics*, 70(2-4), 428-435.

Sutherland, W. J.; Broad, S.; Butchart, S. H.; Clarke, S. J.; Collins, A. M.; Dicks, L. V., y Ockendon, N. (2019). «A horizon scan of emerging issues for global conservation in 2019». *Trends in Ecology & Evolution*, 34(1), 83-94.

Thielens, A.; Bell, D.; Mortimore, D. B.; Greco, M. K.; Martens, L., y Joseph, W. (2018). «Exposure of insects to radio-frequency electromagnetic fields from 2 to 120 ghz». *Sci. Rep.*, 8, 1-10.

Thill, A.; Cammaerts, M. C., y Balmori, A. (2024). «Biological effects of electromagnetic fields on insects: a systematic review and meta-analysis». *Reviews on Environmental Health*, 39(4), 853-869.

Tsai, Y. B.; Liu, J. Y.; Ma, K. F.; Yen, H. Y.; Chen, K. S.; Chen, Y. I., y Lee, C. P. (2006). «Precursory phenomena associated with the 1999 Chi-Chi earthquake in Taiwan as identified under the iSTEP program». *Physics and Chemistry of the Earth, Parts A/B/C*, 31(4-9), 365-377.

Vácha, M.; Půžová, T., y Kvíćalová, M. (2009). «Radio frequency magnetic fields disrupt magnetoreception in American cockroach». *Journal of Experimental Biology*, 212(21), 3473-3477.

Vaitkuvienė, D. y Dagys, M. (2014). «Possible effects of electromagnetic field on White Storks Ciconia ciconia breeding on low-voltage electricity line poles». *Zoology and Ecology*, 24(4), 289-296.

Vaitl, D.; Propson, N.; Stark, R., y Schienle, A. (2001). «Natural very-low-frequency sferics and headache». *Int. J. Biometeorol.*, 45, 115-123.

—; Propson, N.; Stark, R.; Walter, B., y Schienle, A. (2001). «Headache and sferics». *Headache*, 41, 845-853.

Vargová, B.; Kurimský, J.; Cimbala, R.; Kosterec, M.; Majláth, I.; Pipová, N., y Majláthová, V. (2017). «Ticks and radio-frequency signals: behavioural response of ticks (*Dermacentor reticulatus*) in a 900 MHz electromagnetic field». *Systematic and Applied Acarology*, 22(5), 683-693.

Vencloviene, J.; Babarskiene, R.; Slapikas, R., y Sakalyte, G. (2013). «The association between phenomena on the Sun, geomagnetic activity, meteorological variables, and cardiovascular characteristic of patients with myocardial infarction». *International Journal of Biometeorology*, 57(5), 797-804.

Villoresi, G.; Dorman, L. I.; Ptitsyna, N. G.; Iucci, N., y Tyasto, M. I. (1995). «Forbush decreases as indicators of health-hazardous geomagnetic storms». *International Cosmic Ray Conference* (vol. 4, p. 1106).

—; Ptitsyna, N. G.; Tiasto, M. I., y Iucci, N. (1998). «Myocardial infarct and geomagnetic disturbances: analysis of data on morbidity and mortality». *Biofizika*, 43(4), 623-631.

Walach, H.; Betz, H. D., y Schweickhardt, A. (2001). «Sferics and Headache, a prospective study». *Cephalalgia*, 21, 685-690.

Waldmann-Selsam, C.; Balmori-de la Puente, A.; Breunig, H., y Balmori, A. (2016). «Radiofrequency radiation injures trees around mobile phone base stations». *Science of the Total Environment*, 572, 554-569.

Warnke, U. (2007). «Bees, birds and mankind. Destroying nature by "electrosmog"». *Competence Initiative*, 46 pp.

Wang, K.; Chen, Q. F.; Sun, S., y Wang, A. (2006). «Predicting the 1975 Haicheng earthquake». *Bulletin of the Seismological Society of America*, 96(3), 757-795.

Wolf & Wolf (2004). «Increased incidence of cancer near a cell-phone transmitter station». *International Journal of Cancer Prevention*, vol. 1.

Yang, A. C.; Fuh, J. L.; Huang, N. E.; Shia, B. C.; Peng, C. K., y Wang, S. J. (2011). «Temporal associations between weather and headache: analysis by empirical mode decomposition». *PloS one*, 6(1), e14612.

Yokoi, S.; Ikeya, M.; Yagi, T., y Nagai, K. (2003). «Mouse circadian rhythm before the Kobe earthquake in 1995». *Bioelectromagnetics*, 24(4), 289-291.

Zwamborn, A. P.; Vossen, S. H.; Leersum, B. J.; Owens, M. A., y Mäkel, W. N. (2003). *Effects of Global Communication system radio-frequency fields on Well Being and Cognitive Functions of human subjects with and without subjective complaints*. Netherlands Organisation for Applied Scientific Research (TNO).

www.ingramcontent.com/pod-product-compliance
Lightning Source LLC
Chambersburg PA
CBHW031326230926
51848CB00001B/103
9788410354791